CONTENTS

ACKNOWLEDGMENTS

I would like to thank Alice Feinstein, editorial director, for putting her trust in me to write a cookbook that would meet the high standards of Prima Publishing. I also would like to thank my project editor, Michelle McCormack, who not only is wonderful to work with but whose attention to detail and insightful suggestions have once again proven invaluable to me. Thanks to Susan Sugnet, cover designer; and the entire staff at Prima Publishing for their excellent professionalism in bringing this book to publication.

I would especially like to dedicate this book to my husband, Bob. No cookbook of mine would be complete without his constant support, constructive critiques, and his input of innovative ideas; and to my children, David, Adam, and Laura, whose accomplishments continue to be a source of tremendous pride for me.

Special thanks go to many of my friends who enthusiastically shared some of their favorite recipes with me. They are Connie Brothers, Ellie Densen, Sonia Ettinger, Shula Lavie, Joanne Madsen, Katherine Moyers, Judy Neiman, Rosemary Plapp, Susan and Michael Wall, Anita Weiss, and Jo Gail Wenzel.

THE ULTIMATE

LOW-CARB

DIET COOKBOOK

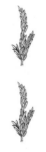

OVER 200 FABULOUS
RECIPES TO ADD
VARIETY AND GREAT
TASTE TO YOUR
LOW-CARBOHYDRATE
LIFESTYLE

Donna Pliner Rodnitzky

PRIMA PUBLISHING

Published by Prima Publishing, Roseville, California. Member of the Crown Publishing Group, a division of Random House, Inc.

PRIMA PUBLISHING and colophon are trademarks of Random House, Inc., registered with the United States Patent and Trademark Office.

A per-serving nutritional breakdown is provided for each recipe. If a range is given for an ingredient amount, the breakdown is based on the smaller number. If a range is given for servings, the breakdown is based on the smaller number. If a choice of ingredients is given in an ingredient listing, the breakdown is calculated using the first choice. Nutritional content may vary depending on the specific brands or types of ingredients used. "Optional" ingredients or those for which no specific amount is stated are not included in the breakdown. Nutritional figures are rounded to the nearest whole number.

Library of Congress Cataloging-in-Publication Data
Rodnitzky, Donna.
  The ultimate low-carb diet cookbook : over 200 fabulous recipes to add variety and great taste to your low-carbohydrate lifestyle / Donna Rodnitzky.
    p.   cm.
  Includes index.
  ISBN 0-7615-3456-3
  1. Low-carbohydrate diet—Recipes. I. Donna Rodnitzky. II. Title.
RM237.73.R63 2001
641.5'638—dc21   2001033171

03 04 DD 10 9 8 7 6 5 4
Printed in the United States of America

First Edition

Visit us online at www.primapublishing.com

INTRODUCTION

In the 1970s, Dr. Robert C. Atkins' book, *Dr. Atkins' Diet Revolution,* revolutionized the way millions of people dieted. Instead of encouraging readers to restrict the amount of fat in their diets, as most other diet experts stressed at that time, Dr. Atkins emphasized reducing the daily intake of refined carbohydrates. He was convinced that carbohydrates were the main culprits leading to weight gain. He reasoned that a diet consisting of sweet foods rich in sugar, or starch-containing foods such as grains, cereals, pasta, and potatoes, causes an increase in the production of insulin, and when there is excessive insulin in our bloodstream, the food we eat is quickly converted into fat.

Just as important, he noted that high-carbohydrate meals leave people feeling unsatisfied and constantly seeking additional ways to curb their hunger. Dr. Atkins' acclaimed theory proposed that by adhering to a low-carbohydrate diet, the resulting decrease in insulin production could reduce conversion to fat and quell the constant sense of hunger, making it easier to lose weight, even when eating a diet that does not strictly limit fats.

Since the introduction of Dr. Atkins' book, several other authors have published books with diet plans focusing on the low-carbohydrate diet. Each emphasizes the need to restrict carbohydrates in the diet, but offers a slight variation on the original Dr. Atkins diet. In chapter 2, I provide an overview of several of these diets to allow you to compare the merits of each individual plan and evaluate which one might be best suited to your lifestyle.

With so many millions of people who are enthusiastic about this approach to dieting, I was delighted to have the opportunity to write *The Ultimate Low-Carb Diet Cookbook*. This collection of more than 200 exciting recipes is designed to appeal to everyone who has made the commitment to reduce the amount of carbohydrates in their diet as a means of losing weight and maintaining a healthier lifestyle.

The Ultimate Low-Carb Diet Cookbook begins with a discussion, in simple terms, of the nature of carbohydrates and their metabolism in order to help you understand the philosophy and science behind the low-carbohydrate approach to dieting. For some of you who are already following this approach, it may not be entirely new information. For those who have been curious about the diet or are contemplating trying it, however, my goal is to present enough basic information to allow you to understand the underlying principles of this approach, and to feel confident about diving in. Readers who desire more than a basic understanding of these nutritional concepts may wish to seek a more definitive scientific description of the low-carbohydrate diet provided in publications by one of the many health professionals with special expertise in human nutrition.

After the discussion of the principles of the low-carbohydrate diet, the remainder of the book features more than 200 recipes that put this philosophy into practice. I hope you will not only savor these recipes, but also use them as an inspiration to create your own low-carbohydrate masterpieces.

Chapter 4, the first recipe chapter, Appetizer Excitement, provides a host of flavorful temptations to share with friends or family. Although snacking should be kept to a minimum while on this diet, there may be times during the day when you need a quick bite to get you to the next meal. It is also great to enjoy a tidbit or two while sharing in good conversation, enjoying television, or watching a movie. So start off the evening with Mushrooms Stuffed with Italian Sausage, Creamy Herb Dip, or Smoked Salmon Mousse—you won't ever be tempted to serve potato chips again.

In Chapter 5, Startling Soups, you will find a wide variety of delicious, satisfying, and healthy low-carbohydrate soups. I personally find that nothing satisfies my appetite faster than a bowl of soup before a meal. While most soups have the added benefit of being warming on a cold, blustery day, the recent popularity of cold soups has introduced a refreshing way to cool down on a hot, sultry day. All of the soups in this book are made with low-carbohydrate ingredients, and you will be both delighted and surprised at the number of ways ordinary ingredients such as zucchini can be transformed into a zestful and creamy textured soup. If you only have time at lunch for a quick bowl of soup, you will be impressed with Curried Cauliflower Soup or Savory Zucchini Soup, both richly flavored and satisfying. When friends are over for a barbecue, serve mugs of Spicy Roasted Red Pepper Soup as you relax on the patio. Let your mantra be "Soups on."

If you are a salad lover, then look no further than my chapter Savvy Salads, containing over 25 recipes for you to enjoy. Salads have been an essential component of a good meal for centuries, but in recent years they have evolved from a simple bowl of greens into a cornucopia of tastes, textures, and colors. With so many fresh salad ingredients now readily available year round in your local supermarket, a modern salad can brim with a surprising variety of novel greens adorned with an enticing array of traditional and exotic vegetables harvested all over the world. With the sprinkling of a zesty vinaigrette, these garden masterpieces can effortlessly be elevated to gourmet heights.

Not only do salads provide a delicious and healthy way of dining, they are also truly satisfying to both the palate and the eye. Just as impressive, with the addition of poultry, meat, seafood, eggs, or cheese, these salads can easily be transformed into main course fare. For example, by adding leftover meats, such as Southwestern Rubbed Flank Steak, to spinach and other salad ingredients, you can create a Savory Spinach Salad with Steak and Blue Cheese, an exceptionally delicious and satisfying main course. Leftover chicken or turkey can be used to create a Cobb salad, or by adding last night's ham, a hearty Chef's Salad can suddenly appear. Whether you only prepare the salad recipes provided in this book or use them as an inspiration for creations of your own, you will discover that salads provide the ultimate opportunity to creatively incorporate healthy, low-carbohydrate foods that complement each other in taste, color, and texture.

Chapter 7, Masterful Main Courses, highlights over 60 delectable recipes to be served at breakfast, lunch, or dinner. Whether you are a novice in the kitchen or a gourmet cook, you will be delighted to discover how easy it is to add variety, and "spice," to your daily low-carbohydrate meal planning. To help you greet the morning with a smile, there is a host of tempting breakfast egg dishes that provide a deliciously satisfying way to start the day. Many of these creations can be assembled quickly in minutes or made ahead. And just as welcoming, most can be refrigerated for a day or two or cut into serving-size portions and frozen. So, instead of fretting over your breakfast choice as you prepare to dash out the door, consider treating yourself to a tasty Mushroom Omelet or a tempting serving of Scrambled Eggs with Smoked Salmon—both are breakfasts of champion dieters.

This chapter also contains a variety of ideas for preparing meat, poultry, and seafood main dishes to tempt you at lunch or dinner. Try Savory Rubbed Baby Back Ribs, a delicious mouthful that gets its zesty flavor from a savory rub that requires only a few minutes to prepare. What's more, by simply making an extra large batch of the rub and storing it in a covered container, you will have enough flavoring left over to rescue dozens of otherwise bland meals. You will be thrilled to discover how this rub or some of the better commercial varieties can magically transform a salmon filet into a culinary sensation or a Cornish hen into a gourmet delight. You will find that rubs are just one of the many ways to add some excitement to mealtime. In this chapter, you also will learn how the simple addition of a few herbs, spices, or a sauce can transform ordinary fare into an instant culinary treat. Try Chipotle Marinated Flank Steak or

Lemon Chicken, both fabulously mouthwatering recipes that belie their simplicity.

Are you a vegetarian? There's plenty here for you as well. You will be delighted with the wide selection of main courses found in this book that meet your needs, and just as pleased to find that many of the recipes that include meat, seafood, or poultry can become newly ordained vegetarian dishes by simply substituting with tofu, tempeh, or even Portobello mushrooms. Whether your tastes run to beef or tofu, as you read this chapter, you will be constantly reminded that being on a low-carbohydrate diet does not mean that mealtime has to be boring.

Even those of us who are not card-carrying vegetarians enjoy a side of vegetables as an accompaniment to a good meal. Although some vegetables are not permitted in a low-carbohydrate diet, I am confident that you will be pleased with the novel recipes I have created using low-carbohydrate vegetables. Chapter 8, Veritable Vegetables, proved to be the greatest challenge for me since so many of our favorite vegetables are forbidden on a low-carbohydrate diet. Who doesn't salivate over French fried potatoes, bourbon-flavored sweet potatoes, or gingered carrots? But the fact is that these foods are forbidden on the diet. My solution to this dilemma was to find more new and imaginative ways to endow low-carbohydrate vegetables with the same flavor and appeal as these forbidden delicacies.

Actually, this mission proved to be quite simple and exciting. Spinach, for example, is not only good for you but is a wonderfully versatile vegetable. It can be eaten raw, served in a delectable salad, or when cooked and combined with other flavorful ingredients, transformed into savory dishes, such as Spinach Custard or Sautéed Spinach with Garlic and Pine Nuts. Even broccoli haters will hold up the white flag after one taste of zesty Broccoli with Garlic and Cheese. Of course, we cannot ignore the venerable zucchini, the vegetable every gardener wants, or needs, to share with friends. Since it grows so bountifully in the garden, there is always a need to find new and better ways to use it. My favorite recipe is Zucchini Soufflé, a dish that receives rave reviews whenever I serve it. After trying some of the more than 35 low-carbohydrate vegetable recipes in this cookbook, you will soon agree that with a little imagination in the kitchen you can derive as much satisfaction from such unlikely gourmet candidates as zucchini and spinach as you might from those "other" vegetables.

The last chapter, Dazzling Desserts, provides recipes for achieving a crowning finish to a meal. Who says you can't have your cake and eat it too! You will find 30 recipes for dessert fare ranging from simple cookies and sweet breads to sumptuous creations that are not only delicious, but also are very low in carbohydrates. Many of these tasteful gems are elegant enough to serve after a candlelight dinner, while others can be enjoyed while relaxing on the patio. Just consider how liberated you will feel compared to your frustration on all the diets that won't even allow you a tiny taste of anything associated with that forbidden word "dessert." So, whether you are craving Crème Brûlée, Ultimate Cheesecake, or a slice of a Hazelnut Cake Roll, you no longer have to leave the table feeling deprived of a dessert or guilty that you ate one. Let the party begin and enjoy it from start to finish with a richly deserved dessert.

If what you crave is ease in preparation, luscious flavors, and variety in the low-carbohydrate foods you eat, this book is for you. I hope you will be as eager to try these recipes as I was excited in creating them, and that *The Ultimate Low-Carb Diet Cookbook* will become your "ultimate" resource for delicious and healthy low-carbohydrate dining. Whether you are preparing a delicious meal for your family or a sumptuous offering for your most discerning guests, I am confident that this book will enable you to present mealtime masterpieces with pride. Most of all, I hope it will add the culinary variety that you crave and provide the stimulus to make the low-carbohydrate diet a healthy and satisfying way of life.

part one

LEARNING

chapter one

DEFINING THE LOW-CARBOHYDRATE DIET
It's Not Rocket Science

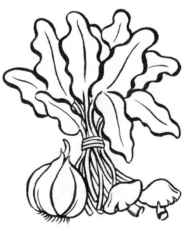

UNDERSTANDING THE METABOLIC AND nutritional principles behind the low-carbohydrate diet is not rocket science, but without an adequate discussion, outlined in simple terms, it can seem that way. There are only a few simple definitions that you need to familiarize yourself with in order to understand clearly the scientific theory behind the diet and how it allows you to lose weight in an easy and healthful way. So, before delving into the explanation, let's define those few terms that will set you on the pathway to becoming a first-class carbomeister:

- **Calorie:** Officially a measure of heat, a calorie, in dietary terms, is a measure of the amount of energy the body can derive from a particular food. The more calories provided by a foodstuff, the longer it will take the body to "burn up" that nutrient.

- **Carbohydrate:** Carbohydrates are one of three major nutrient groups that provide energy for the body, the other two being protein and fat. All carbohydrates are composed of single sugars or strings of sugar bound together. Single sugars, such as table sugar (sucrose), fruit sugar (fructose), and dairy sugar (lactose), are referred to as simple carbohydrates. In plants, stored sugars are bound together, resulting in complex carbohydrates, often referred to as starches. Most complex carbohydrates, such as potato starch or wheat flour, are edible and digestible, but some, such as cellulose (from celery), cannot be digested.

- **Glucagon:** Glucagon is one of two major hormones produced by the pancreas (the other is insulin). When the blood sugar level is low, glucagon is released and acts to stimulate the liver to break down its stored glycogen into glucose and release it into the bloodstream. This hormone also promotes the breakdown of protein and fat to produce energy when blood glucose is not at an adequate level for the body's needs.

- **Glucose:** Glucose (also known as dextrose) is a simple sugar found in fruits and honey. It is also the form of sugar that circulates in the human bloodstream. The blood level of glucose is the major stimulus for insulin secretion.

- **Glycogen:** Glycogen is the form in which the body stores excess glucose in the liver and muscles. It is essentially composed of a number of glucose molecules strung together. Glycogen is an energy storehouse for the body and, when needed, can be broken down into glucose and released from its storage sites.

- **Insulin:** Insulin is one of two major hormones produced by the pancreas (the other is glucagon). The pancreas releases it when the blood glucose rises. Insulin then helps transfer glucose into cells, where it can be used as a source of energy. In fatty tissue, insulin promotes the conversion of excess glucose to fat, and in the liver, it causes excess glucose to be stored as glycogen. In muscle, it promotes the entry of amino acids, the building blocks of protein. The medical condition diabetes is due to inadequate production of insulin, reduced sensitivity to its effects, or both. Under some circumstances, insulin elevates cholesterol levels and inhibits the breakdown of previously stored fat.

- **Ketones:** Ketones are chemicals resulting from the breakdown of fat that occurs when the body does not have enough glucose for energy production and the liver's store of glycogen has been used up. Although there are always some ketones circulating in the bloodstream, fasting or a very low-carbohydrate diet increases the amount of these substances, creating a condition referred to as *ketosis*.

With these definitions in mind, how does the low-carbohydrate diet work? In the simplest terms, the body's response to a carbohydrate meal is to secrete insulin while at the same time suppressing release of the other pancreatic hormone, glucagon. As we age, excessive insulin secretion can occur in response to even ordinary amounts of carbohydrates in the diet because of "insulin resistance," a condition in which our cells respond subnormally to the hormone, requiring the pancreas to secrete more of it just to achieve a normal effect. One of the basic underlying principles of the low-carbohydrate diet is that insulin (especially excessive insulin) has potentially negative health effects while the opposite is true for glucagon. After a high-carbohydrate meal, insulin tries to store the excess glucose derived from the meal as glycogen in the liver and muscles. As this storage capacity is limited and easily saturated, insulin next turns to fat as a storage vehicle for the remaining glucose. Not only does excess insulin promote the deposition of fat in this way, it also may have other negative health effects, such as elevation of blood cholesterol and retention of fluid and salt.

chapter two

THE LOWDOWN ON LOW-CARBOHYDRATE DIETS

Choose the Plan That's Best for You

* * * * * * * * * *

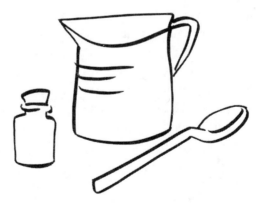

* * * * * * * * * *

THE OVERWHELMING POPULARITY OF low-carbohydrate diets began in the 1960s and 1970s, when Dr. Robert C. Atkins' diet made its debut, along with other similar plans, such as the Stillman diet and the Scarsdale diet. Millions of people soon discovered how easy it was to adhere to a low-carbohydrate diet regimen in order to lose unwanted pounds successfully and keep them off. While each of these diet plans has an exclusive weight loss regimen, what is most striking is the common thread that runs through all of them: the restriction of daily carbohydrate intake in order to keep insulin production to a minimum. To achieve this goal, each of these diets suggests increasing the daily intake of protein by utilizing a menu concentrating on such foods as eggs, meat, fish, and a variety of cheeses and dairy products.

Despite the opinion of some medical researchers in the 1980s disputing the benefits of a low-carbohydrate diet, most of these diet plans continue to be very popular today. Although experts agreed that weight loss could be achieved with this strategy, some scientists expressed concern about other health risks that might result from following low-carbohydrate guidelines. Some of these experts promoted the benefits of a minimal-fat diet. They strongly believed that this approach was much healthier than a diet rich in protein and fat. Acceptable foods allowed in the minimal-fat diet included carbohydrate-rich items, such as pasta, rice, bread, grains, and fruits. Other foods, such as eggs, red meat, and butter, were strictly "taboo" and were deemed unhealthful. This new dietary regimen was quickly endorsed by the media and nutritionists and ultimately by the government as reflected in its Food Pyramid Guideline. The premise of the pyramid is that the greatest health benefit is derived from consuming foods found at the bottom of the pyramid, such as breads, pasta, cereal, rice, grains, fruits, and vegetables—in other words, foods rich in carbohydrates. Conversely, the guideline recommended that foods such as meats and dairy products be severely limited and that fats and oil be eaten sparingly.

By the 1990s, a number of medical experts began to publicly acknowledge the basic failure experienced by many people attempting to lose weight while following this extremely restrictive minimal-fat diet. It was becoming clear that despite the Establishment's endorsement of this diet, a great number of Americans were still overweight, and, worse, extreme obesity was on the rise. You might ask how people could be getting fatter when they were eating less fat.

After years of people following the experts who claimed that the only way to lose weight healthfully was to reduce drastically the amount of dietary fat consumed, it appeared that this logic didn't apply to everyone, and many could not successfully lose weight on such a diet. A different breed of experts then introduced totally new rules of engagement for the battle against the bulging midriff. They told us that eating fat doesn't necessarily make you fat and that it may be hard to lose weight by limiting calories alone. Even more important, they recognized that very few of us can adhere to a diet that is too restrictive and allows no choice. These low-carb gurus are the authors of the diet plans I describe in the following discussion.

As you read the brief summaries I have provided of a few of the currently popular low-carbohydrate diets, you will be pleased to find that most of the diet plans can be followed with little effort and without too much intrusion on your valuable time. Although a donut or a muffin makes for a quick breakfast, with a little planning, a delicious egg creation can be prepared ahead, refrigerated or frozen, and then be ready to heat up in the same amount of time it takes to toast a bagel. You also will be delighted to discover that eating at your favorite restaurant does not need to be a guilt-ridden trip. If you love pizza, you will soon discover that you can feel just as satisfied eating the topping without the crust. The same can be said for a slice of heavenly cheesecake.

In the final analysis, your devotion will be richly rewarded when you find that you are not only able to enjoy a healthy life but you can dine out with friends or host a traditional holiday dinner and lose weight at the same time.

Low-Carbohydrate Diets in a Nutshell

The popularity of the low-carbohydrate diet has generated a variety of diet plans authored by leading health authorities. I have provided here brief summaries of some of the most popular published low-carbohydrate diets. As you read through these summaries, I hope it will stimulate you to browse through several of the diet plan books on your own and choose the diet best suited for you.

Robert C. Atkins, M.D., *Dr. Atkins' New Diet Revolution* (Avon, 1992)

Dr. Atkins' diet is essentially a high-protein/low-carbohydrate diet plan based on a lifetime nutritional philosophy. The emphasis is on the consumption of "nutrient-dense" unprocessed foods, along with vita-nutrient supplements, including a full-spectrum multivitamin and an essential oils/fatty acid formula. Foods that are restricted in this diet include all processed/refined carbohydrates, such as high-sugar foods, pasta, breads, cereal, and all starchy vegetables.

Dr. Atkins' theory is that high-carbohydrate foods cause your body to increase its production of insulin. High insulin levels result in conversion of excess carbohydrates into body fat. He also believes that high-carbohydrate foods leave you feeling less satisfied than those containing adequate amounts of fat. Due to this unsatisfied feeling, you eat more, and, what's worse, additional insulin is released and you get hungry again sooner.

The Atkins plan starts with a 14-Day Induction Diet, which is intended to correct an unbalanced metabolism. The induction phase requires that your daily carbohydrate intake not exceed 20 grams, an extreme restriction that is designed to induce *ketosis*. Ketosis involves the breakdown of fat to provide energy. By restricting daily carbohydrates to 20 grams or less, the body must utilize its stored carbohydrates. The daily carbohydrate intake is quickly used up and the body turns to stored fat as a source of energy. Through all this, Dr. Atkins reminds us that when fewer carbohydrates are consumed, the body will naturally produce less insulin.

The next phase is the Ongoing Weight Loss Diet, which is more lenient than the Induction phase. You are allowed to increase your daily carbohydrate intake by up to 5 grams. This level of increased carbohydrate intake can be maintained for one or more weeks, after which an additional 5 grams of daily carbohydrate intake can be added. As you continue to add more carbohydrates, after a variable period of weeks, an individual will eventually reach his or her critical carbohydrate level for losing, or CCLL. At this level of carbohydrate intake, you will not lose any more weight; above this level, you will begin to put on pounds. Once you have identified your own CCLL and have only 5 to 10 pounds remaining to lose, you begin Pre-Maintenance. These last few remaining pounds should come off slowly, so the goal is to adjust daily carbohydrate consumption to a level where you are losing less than a pound per week. Ultimately, you will arrive at your *ideal weight* and be ready for the Maintenance Diet, Dr. Atkins' strategy for keeping the pounds off.

Richard F. Heller, M.A., Ph.D., and Rachael F. Heller, M.A., Ph.D., *The Carbohydrate Addict's LifeSpan Program* (Dutton, 1998)

This is one of several books the Hellers have written on the subject of low-carbohydrate dieting. The Carbohydrate Addict's diet is intended to be very user friendly and simple to follow. On this program, you do not have to count calories, measure your food, or worry about food exchanges. Despite this liberal approach, the Hellers promise that following their prescribed guidelines will normalize elevated blood insulin levels that are responsible for your cravings and your weight gain.

The Hellers stress that their program is personalized to fit your needs, your preferences, and your lifestyle since it presents you with options that you can choose from to lose weight. They point out that the fact that their program is not rigid but, rather, completely adaptable makes it easier to stay with. If you are hungry, then you can eat more. You also can eat out and even indulge in a fancy dessert—all without guilt. The important thing the Hellers stress is to learn "how" to eat the foods you desire, so that you will have the freedom to choose when, where, what, and how much you want in order to be satisfied.

The Carbohydrate Addict's diet plan consists of two essential parts: the Program's Basic Plan and the Options for Life. These two components are meant to balance and complement each other. The Basic Plan of the diet incorporates three guidelines that are essential to help you reduce your cravings and lose weight. These three guidelines must be followed strictly for two weeks. Within a few days, you should see a dramatic decrease or elimination of your cravings, and after two weeks, you should be able to calculate your weekly weight loss. At this time, you select options from the Options for Life part of the program.

The three guidelines of the initial Basic Plan are:

1. Eat a balanced reward meal every day.

The doctors give you something to look forward to each day. Once a day, they allow you to treat yourself to a reward meal containing carbohydrate-rich foods, such as starches, snack foods, or sweets that you crave. It is suggested that the reward meal start with 2 cups of fresh salad with dressing, followed by one-third craving-reducing protein, one-third craving-reducing vegetable, and one-third carbohydrate-rich foods (including dessert). The Hellers do not require that you weigh or measure the food you eat, but the thirds of food should be equal in portion size. If you are still hungry after having finished the reward meal, you are allowed to go back for more as long as you maintain the equal-sized portion of every component of the meal; that is, you cannot splurge for seconds on dessert alone. *Balance* is the key factor in the reward meal.

2. Complete your reward meal within one hour.

The Hellers stress that after eating carbohydrate-rich foods, insulin is released in two waves. The first wave of insulin release occurs within a few minutes of eating, and the amount released is predetermined by how much and how often you have eaten carbohydrate-rich foods during the past day. If your body has become accustomed to carbohydrate-rich foods, it will expect each new meal or snack to be just as rich in carbohydrates and may release a greater amount of insulin than necessary in this first wave. By restricting most of your carbohydrate-rich foods to a once-a-day reward meal, this excessive insulin release mechanism is less likely to be triggered by your current meal.

The doctors go on to explain that the second wave of insulin release depends on how much carbohydrate-rich food is included in the current meal. This wave is released over time, peaking at about 70 minutes, so that if a meal can be finished before that time, this portion of insulin released can be prevented from reaching its peak.

3. Eat only craving-reducing foods at all other meals and snacks.

The Hellers define craving-reducing foods as high-fiber vegetables and protein-rich foods. In their plan, all meals and snacks, except for the reward meal, should be well balanced and mostly comprised of these high-fiber and protein-rich choices.

After two weeks on the Basic Plan, you are ready to add the next phase of The Carbohydrate Addict's diet: Options for Life. A variety of options are available, including an exercise program, reducing caffeine intake, and adding chromium to your diet, just to name a few. In a nutshell, the options are designed to allow some latitude in finding ways to reduce your insulin levels further and promote effortless weight loss.

Michael R. Eades, M.D., and Mary Dan Eades, M.D., *Protein Power* (Bantam, 1996)

The gist of *Protein Power* is that you can reduce cholesterol and triglyceride levels in your bloodstream, lose body fat, lower your blood pressure, and normalize your blood sugar simply by changing your diet.

While the emphasis is on including enough protein in your diet, the Eades pay a great deal of attention to the role that excess insulin and insulin resistance play in creating a multitude of metabolic disorders. As important as insulin is, they also point out the critical role in this nutritional drama played by its counterpart, the hormone glucagon. The Eades explain that when we eat, insulin is what drives our metabolism to store excess food energy to be used later when needed. Conversely, glucagon is the hormone that drives metabolism in the opposite direction, letting us burn our stored fat for needed energy. In short, insulin's major responsibility is to keep the blood sugar level from rising too high while glucagon acts to prevent the blood sugar level from falling too low. The Eades believe that the diet they have developed maximizes the release of glucagon and, at the same time, minimizes the release of insulin.

The Protein Power Program includes several important guidelines, all of which are carefully explained in their book. I list only two of them here to give you an idea of what the diet entails:

1. Determine your protein needs.

To determine your protein needs, you must first calculate your lean body mass, according to a detailed formula fully explained in the book. The information gleaned from this calculation becomes the basis for determining the minimum amount of daily high-quality complete protein you need. Once you calculate your daily protein requirements, your meal plan revolves around this prescribed amount. Each of your three daily meals should include at least the prescribed amount of protein and include such foods as fish, red meat, poultry, low-fat cheese (feta, cottage, Muenster, and mozzarella), eggs, and tofu. On this diet, it is acceptable to have several snacks during the day when hungry, and the plan suggests that each snack contain an amount of protein equal to half of a protein meal serving.

2. Add carbohydrate grams.

Individuals who need to lose a lot of fat and/or correct a health problem are advised to include 30 carbohydrate grams or less divided over the day. For those who only need to lose a little fat, recompose their lean-to-fat ratio, or simply improve their general health, the Eades feel it is permissible to include 55 carbohydrate grams per day.

Beyond these important guidelines, the Protein Power diet suggests that you aim for 25 grams of fiber in your diet each day, that you choose healthy fats, and, above all, that you never let yourself get hungry.

Barry Sears, Ph.D., *The Zone* (HarperCollins, 1995)

Dr. Sears defines the Zone as the metabolic state in which your body works at peak efficiency. In order to get into the Zone, he believes that you must learn to treat food as if it were a powerful drug. Using colorful analogies, Dr. Sears likens eating food to a continuous intravenous drip—it must be eaten in a controlled fashion and in proper proportions.

Dr. Sears acknowledges that some carbohydrates are needed in our diet, but the important question he poses is how much is *some* and how much is *too much?* The book answers these questions in great detail. Like many of the other experts, Dr. Sears emphasizes that too many carbohydrates means too much insulin, and, in his scheme, too much insulin takes you out of the Zone.

This book proceeds to discuss the *glycemic index,* a measure of the rate at which carbohydrates enter the bloodstream. Some carbohydrates, such as simple sugars, enter the bloodstream at a much more rapid rate than others. Eating too many of these high-glycemic carbohydrates results in an excessive release of insulin, which encourages the storage of fat.

With this information in hand, let's quickly review how Dr. Sears recommends that you get into the Zone. He believes that every meal and snack you eat should have the desired balance of macronutrients—protein, carbohydrates, and fat—in order to produce a favorable hormonal response. As discussed below, Dr. Sears makes specific recommendations as to the amount of each of these macronutrients that should be included in the ideal diet:

The Lowdown on Low-Carbohydrate Diets
····

PROTEIN   In Dr. Sears' diet plan, your daily protein requirement depends on your weight, your percentage of body fat, and your level of physical activity. The book provides a detailed formula on how to determine your protein requirement. You then divide that amount of protein evenly over the three meals and two snacks allowed each day. Dr. Sears suggests that you think of your total protein requirement as a sum of protein blocks, with each block consisting of 7 grams of protein. For example, if your total protein requirement is 70 grams, that would constitute 10 protein blocks of 7 grams each.

CARBOHYDRATES   Once you have calculated your protein requirement, the Sears plan suggests that one carbohydrate block (each containing about 9 grams of carbohydrates) be consumed for every protein block. The kind of carbohydrate you eat is very important. On this diet, it is essential that you emphasize low-glycemic carbohydrates, such as those found in fiber-rich fruits and vegetables. In addition, it is important to avoid foods such as bread, grains, pasta, potatoes, corn, and any high-glycemic fruits and vegetables, such as bananas, papayas, and carrots.

FATS   A Zone-favorable meal includes fat. The kind of fat you include is very important, however. This plan advises that you severely restrict arachidonic acid, a fat found in egg yolks, organ meats, and fatty red meats. Additionally, saturated fats found in animal sources and dairy products should be kept to a minimum. "Good" fats are the monounsaturated variety found in olive oil, canola oil, macadamia nuts, olives, and avocados. As is the case with carbohydrates in this diet, for every protein block you consume, the plan recommends that you add one fat block.

H. Leighton Steward, Morrison C. Bethea, M.D., Sam S. Andrews, M.D., and Luis A. Balart, M.D., *Sugar Busters!* (Ballantine, 1998)

Like its low-carbohydrate brethren, the goal of the Sugar Busters! diet is the modulation of insulin. The developers of this diet agree that to prevent excessive insulin release it is vital to control the intake of sugar. Their emphasis is on selecting foods that stimulate insulin secretion in a more controlled manner rather than those that cause an immediate outpouring of the hormone.

Carbohydrates are the central theme of this diet since sugar is the basic building block of all carbohydrates. When you eat refined sugars, they are immediately absorbed in a concentrated fashion, resulting in a rapid secretion of large quantities of insulin. Conversely, unrefined carbohydrates, as found in fruits, dried beans, whole grains, and green vegetables, require further digestion before absorption. As a result, they cause a proportionately slower rate and lower quantity of insulin secretion.

This diet advocates avoiding refined carbohydrates and encourages consumption of lean meats. The emphasis is on lean because this kind of meat provides the needed protein building blocks of the body without an excessive, uninvited amount of animal fat. Still, the authors point out that there are other important reasons to include adequate amounts of protein in a diet. When protein is ingested, it stimulates the pancreas to secrete the hormone glucagon, which in turn promotes the breakdown of stored body fat.

In summary, the primary goal of this diet is to influence positively the secretion of insulin and glucagon through nutrition. *Sugar Busters!* instructs us that we can easily accomplish this by consuming a diet comprised of natural unrefined sugars, whole unprocessed grains, fruits, vegetables, fiber, and lean meats in proper proportions.

chapter three

A Few Low-Carbohydrate Basics
A How-To for Low-Carb Diets

* * * * * * * * * *

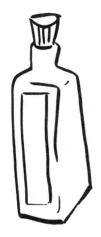

* * * * * * * * *

N OW THAT YOU HAVE read the explanation of the low-carbohydrate diet provided in chapter 2, and been introduced to the currently popular diets, you are ready to become converted to this exciting way of dining or, if already converted, to exclaim a few hallelujahs. After sifting through these chapters, you now recognize that the common thread running through all of these diets is the requirement to restrict the daily consumption of all foods that are high in carbohydrates. While this may sound like an easy feat for most of us to accomplish, for some, it is not.

Many Americans blithely continue on a diet that could include 300 grams or more of carbohydrates per day. This dietary orientation is reinforced by popular guidelines, such as the widely quoted Food Pyramid Guideline, which emphasizes foods rich in carbohydrates, such as breads, pastas, cereals, grains, fruits, and vegetables. The same guideline discourages inclusion of meats and dairy products. However, many of us have found that it is difficult to adhere to this dietary approach, and what's worse, it is hard for most individuals to lose weight in this way. It requires a new mind-set to believe that a steak is acceptable for dinner and mashed potatoes are not, but once you make this leap, the rewards can be impressive.

No matter what low-carbohydrate diet you choose, your ultimate goal will be a lifetime commitment to limiting your daily intake of carbohydrates. Many leading authorities on this subject have published their own guides to the low-carbohydrate foods allowed on their specific diet plans. These are the safest and most practical guides to follow and should be your ultimate resource. Once you have reviewed the foods that have the Low-Carbohydrate Seal of Approval, the next step is to remove, if possible, all those tempting high-carbohydrate foods that are lurking in your pantry and refrigerator. Realizing that everyone in your household may not be following this diet may make this task more difficult to accomplish. If there is any way to separate or discard any of these forbidden foods, though, you will discover how much easier it is to remain true to your low-carbohydrate pledge. Once your cupboard is bare and these forbidden foods are out of sight (and out of mind), the available space is ready to be occupied by a wide variety of other foods that are allowed on the diet. By stocking your larder with an ample supply of the low-carbohydrate foods that are available, you will be ready to prepare a satisfying meal on demand.

In this chapter, I hope to acquaint you with the wide variety of foods that are "legal" in most low-carbohydrate diet plans and used throughout this cookbook. You will learn how to look for these food items in the supermarket, as well as how to prepare and store those that need extra attention. As further help in this new adventure, you will find a general discussion of basic kitchen equipment, as well as a list of cooking terms that you will come across in many of the recipes found in this book.

A Word about Low-Carbohydrate Ingredients

The recipes in this cookbook are as varied and satisfying as they are low in carbohydrates. You will find a wide range of ingredients, from crisp greens to succulent red meat and from rich chocolates to exotic spices. This section was fashioned to acquaint you with some of these foods and to help you select the best ingredients possible for preparing your low-carbohydrate meals.

While weight loss and reducing carbohydrate intake are your ultimate goals, you may find that some of the ingredients listed here and throughout the book are higher in fat or calories than you would prefer. You also may find that certain food items allowed in one of the published diet plans may not be allowed in the others. For example, Dr. Robert C. Atkins recommends excluding milk from your diet while other diets allow it. To solve one of these dilemmas, keep in mind that a majority of low-carbohydrate ingredients can be interchanged with others that also are low in fat or calories. Based on your lifestyle and the particular diet plan you have chosen, you should feel free to make these substitutions as long as the carbohydrate count remains the same.

Stocking the Pantry

The first order of business is to stock your pantry with those essential foodstuffs you will want to have readily available. Later, we will fill the refrigerator. The suggested ingredients are only meant to be a blueprint for the great variety of low-carbohydrate ingredients available for preparing exciting, novel, and mouth-watering dishes:

> **Almond flour:** Almond flour is made from blanched or toasted almonds that have been ground to a fine powder. As almonds are low in carbohydrates, this flour makes an excellent substitute for all-purpose flour. There are a number of sources for almond flour on the Web; simply conduct a search using the words *almond flour*. I bought my almond flour from:
>
> > G & P Ranch
> > P.O. Box 77793
> > Stockton, CA 95267
> > www.almondsonline.com
>
> **Anchovies:** An anchovy is a small fish belonging to the herring family. Fresh anchovies have a delicate flavor, but they are usually purchased in their preserved form, pickled in brine or oil. This method develops their flavor and enhances the zest they bring to a garnish or when added to a main dish. Anchovies are commonly packed in 2-ounce cans as fillets or wrapped around a caper. They are found in the canned fish section of most supermarkets.
>
> **Capers:** Capers are the unopened flower buds of the Mediterranean caper bush. They are preserved, or cured in salt or brine, and then packed in vinegar or salt. As a garnish or condiment, capers add

piquancy to any dish. Capers are found in the olive section of the supermarket.

Chinese Five Spice powder: This spice is a mixture of cloves, cinnamon, fennel, star anise, and Szechwan peppercorns. Chinese Five Spice powder can be found in the spice section of many supermarkets and in Asian food shops.

Darrell Lea Sugar Free Milk Chocolate: This gourmet sugar-free chocolate is made of the finest ingredients by Darrell Lea Chocolate Shops of Australia. It is pure chocolate with no carbohydrates. You can order this fantastic treat online at: www.lowcarboutfitters.com.

Fines Herbs: This seasoning is a combination of parsley, chives, chervil, and tarragon. Fines Herbs can be found in the spice section of most supermarkets.

High-gluten flour: High-gluten flour is wheat flour with the starch and bran removed. There are different high-gluten flours available, so be sure to read the label to assure that the brand you are purchasing yields 75 percent protein and with only 6 grams of carbohydrates per ¼ cup. High-gluten flour is available in most health food stores or in the health section of most supermarkets. There are also a number of sources for buying it on the Web. Enter the word *gluten* or *high-gluten flour.*

Kalamata olives: These glossy black, almond-shaped olives are cured in red wine vinegar, which gives them a salty-sweet taste. Kalamata olives are available by the pound at most specialty food stores or delis. They also can be found in jars or plastic containers in the gourmet or olive section of many supermarkets.

Mayonnaise: A basic French sauce, mayonnaise is an emulsion of raw egg yolks, vegetable oil, spices, and vinegar or lemon juice. It is frequently used as a salad dressing as well as a base for a number of compound sauces. Once you open a jar of mayonnaise, be sure to refrigerate it.

Mirin (rice wine): A golden cooking wine with a sweet and syrupy taste, Mirin is made from sake (Japanese rice wine), sweet rice, and rice malt. The alcohol content of Mirin evaporates during the cooking process, leaving a distinct sweetness. This product is found in the Asian section of many supermarkets and in Asian food shops.

Oils: Oils are a critical ingredient in vinaigrettes or marinades in many low-carbohydrate recipes. In addition, they are frequently the preferred means of cooking because of their lower fat content than butter or shortening. Among the wide variety of oils available, a discussion of the most commonly used ones will help you in your selection:

• *Canola oil:* This oil is made from the seeds of the rape plant. Canola oil has steadily been gaining in popularity due to its healthful profile, which includes a very low saturated fat content, a higher monounsaturated fat content than all other oils except olive oil, and the presence of omega-3 fatty acids.

• *Olive oil:* This classic gourmet ingredient is available in several grades and in various colors. The greener olive oils usually are pressed from greener olives earlier in the season. The labels "extra virgin," "superfine virgin," and "pure" refer to the level of acidity found in the final product. The traditional method of producing olive oil begins by crushing washed and rinsed olives between two very large revolving stone wheels. This process results in a most unpleasant-looking mush, which is then spread on layers of porous mats and subjected to pressure that causes the oil to drip off. The pressure is applied very slowly and steadily to prevent any friction that might produce heat and alter the properties of the new oil. It is this crucial first step that gave rise to the terms "cold pressed" or "first run."

Extra virgin olive oil is the product of the first pressing of the highest quality olives and contains 1 percent or less acid. The finest extra virgin olive oils have less than 1 percent acid. The mashy pulp left over from the first pressing is then mixed with hot water (or chemicals) and processed to make second and third pressed oils. Examples of these oils are *superfine virgin olive oil,* which can have up to 1.5 percent acid; *fine* or *regular virgin,* which ranges from 1.5 to 3 percent; and *virgin* or *pure olive oil,* which has up to 4 percent acidity.

Pure olive oil usually is made from a second pressing and is frequently extracted with chemical solvents and heat. This product has a less pleasant taste. Pure olive oil should be reserved for cooking only and not used as an ingredient in sauces or dressings. All olive oils should be stored in a dark, cool cupboard or in a dark glass or tin.

• *Sesame oil:* There are two varieties of sesame oil. The first, pressed from raw white sesame seeds, is pale yellow in color and has a mild taste. I prefer Asian sesame oil, which is pressed from roasted sesame seeds. This aromatic variety is amber or rich orange in color and has a very distinctive nutty flavor. To keep sesame oil from turning rancid, it is best to refrigerate the bottle once it has been opened. Sesame oil can be found in the Asian section of many supermarkets and health food stores and in Asian food stores.

• *Walnut oil:* This strong-flavored oil is frequently used in France. The imported cold-pressed variety has the best flavor. After you open a bottle of walnut oil, be sure to refrigerate it. Walnut oil is available in health food stores and gourmet shops.

Peppercorns: Like coarse salt and sea salt, peppercorns freshly ground in a pepper mill add a defining flavor to most foods. I have two pepper mills, one for grinding white peppercorns and another for the black variety. Although most of us are more familiar with black pepper, there are some recipes in which white pepper works as well or better since it is less pungent than the black form and is less likely to change the appearance of the other ingredients. Peppercorns can be found in the spice section of most supermarkets, health food stores, and gourmet shops.

A Few Low-Carbohydrate Basics

••••

Pepperoncini: These peppers are green at first, then turn red when allowed to ripen. After the peppers are harvested in the green stage, they usually are pickled. Crunchy and spicy pickled pepperonici are ideal as a garnish, as an addition to a salad, or as an ingredient on an antipasto platter. Pepperonici are found in the olive or pickle section of many supermarkets.

Pine nuts (pignolias or piñon nuts): Pine nuts are small edible seeds found in the cones of the Mediterranean stone pine tree. They can be eaten raw but, when toasted, have a wonderful nutty flavor. Pine nuts can be found in health food stores or in the gourmet section of many supermarkets.

Pork rinds: Pork rinds are deep-fried chunks of pork skin. These versatile snacks will satisfy most cravings for something crispy to eat, as well as delight your taste buds. They are available in a variety of flavors, such as hot and spicy, barbecue, and lemon, just to name a few. Pork rinds can be dipped into guacamole or salsa, used as a topping or filler when crumbled, or even substituted for croutons in your favorite soup or salad. It may be hard to believe, but these tasty morsels are very high in protein and low in carbohydrates. Pork rinds can be found in the snack food section of most supermarkets.

Salt: Once you have tasted foods seasoned with coarse (Kosher) salt, you will never go back to using table salt again. Coarse salt is processed without additives. It can add a gourmet touch by enhancing the flavor of each individual ingredient in a recipe. Another useful salt variety is *fine* sea salt, which is an excellent choice for use in a marinade. If you prefer coarse sea salt, you will need a salt grinder. As both the Kosher and sea varieties are less salty than the iodized form, you may discover that you need more when seasoning your special dish. These salts are available in the spice section of many supermarkets, health food stores, or gourmet shops.

Sriracha hot chili sauce: Sriracha is a hot chili sauce made from serrano chiles, which are the hottest chiles commonly available. It is milder and thicker than other hot pepper sauces. It can be found in the Asian section of many supermarkets and in Asian food shops.

Sweeteners: There are a number of sugar substitutes on the market, and not all are equal in taste and performance. The two that I prefer to use are stevia and Splenda No-Calorie Sweetener. My first choice of sweeteners is Splenda, which is the brand name for sucralose. Sucralose is a sweetening ingredient considered safe by the United States Food and Drug Administration and by the Joint FAO (Food and Agriculture Organization)/WHO (World Health Organization) Expert Committee on Food Additives for everyone to consume. Although Splenda is made from sugar and tastes like sugar, its chemical structure prevents it from being absorbed by the body. Moreover, unlike sugar, it cannot be broken down and utilized for energy in the body. Another kudo for this remarkable sweetener is that it does not have any bitter aftertaste. Splenda is now available in packets (one packet equals 2 teaspoons granulated sugar) or in granular form in most supermarkets. If you cannot find it, or find a store that will order it for you, consider looking on the Internet at online sources (splenda.com, sucralose.com, or lowcarboutfitters.com).

Stevia, frequently referred to as "the sweet herb of Paraguay," is an herb in the chrysanthemum family that grows wild as a small shrub in parts of Paraguay and Brazil. The glycosides in its leaves account for its natural sweetness and are reputed to be 300 times sweeter than sugar. In fact, 1 teaspoon of dried stevia leaves is sweeter than a cup of sugar. As stevia is not absorbed by the body, it has virtually no calories or carbohydrates. Furthermore, it does not affect blood sugar levels. Some people find that it has a bitter aftertaste while others are very pleased with its ability to sweeten certain foods. Stevia is sold as a flavor enhancer in a variety of forms, including liquid and powder form. While it enhances the flavor of certain foods, as in dairy or fruit recipes, stevia is not an acceptable substitute for sugar in baking. Unlike sugar, it does not caramelize and will not add texture, soften a batter, or enhance the browning of most baked goods. Similar to Splenda, there are a number of sources for ordering stevia online. Stevia also is available in most health food stores.

Vanilla protein whey powder: Vanilla whey protein powder is a protein drink containing only 7 grams of carbohydrates per cup. This excellent source of protein powder is a wonderful substitute for flour. You can buy it online (enter the words *vanilla protein whey powder*). It also is available at GNC or many health food stores and in the health section of most supermarkets.

Zero-Carb chocolate chips: As the name implies, these sugar-free chocolate chips have zero carbs. They are packaged in 8-ounce bags. The chocolate chips can be purchased online: www.lowcarboutfitters .com. You also will be interested to know that this company has a multitude of other low-carbohydrate products, such as pasta, cereal, and bread mixes, just to name a few.

What's in the Refrigerator?

Many critical ingredients of low-carbohydrate recipes are perishable and must be kept in the refrigerator. This is especially true of a variety of fresh herbs and other low-carbohydrate, flavor-enhancing ingredients. By selecting the freshest ingredients and properly storing them, you can be assured that each one's unique flavor will be enjoyed to its fullest extent:

Cilantro: Cilantro, also known as Chinese parsley or fresh coriander, is one of the most popular herbs in the world. When we speak of *cilantro,* we are referring to the leaves and stem of the coriander plant while the term *coriander* usually refers to the entire plant, which includes its seeds, stems, roots, flowers, and leaves, all of which are edible. Cilantro is a member of the carrot/parsley family and has a very intense and pungent flavor. When buying cilantro, look for bunches that have crisp, green leaves and an aromatic fragrance.

Avoid those with damaged leaves. Cilantro is found in the produce section of most supermarkets.

Fresh herbs: Fresh herbs are a wonderful way to enhance the flavors of most foods. Although the dried variety is more readily available, easier to use, and requires no preparation, you will find that the flavoring of foods is appreciably more intense when you use fresh herbs.

As some herbs, such as basil, cilantro, tarragon, chervil, and dill, are fragile, they may require more attention. First, remove any rubber bands from these fresh plants. Next, cut off the root ends and lower part of the stems because they draw moisture from the fragile leaves. Once trimmed, loosely wrap the herbs in a damp paper towel and put them in a large enough plastic bag so the leaves and stems will not be crushed. Place the herbs on the top shelf of your refrigerator and use them within a few days. If the herbs need washing before use, simply immerse them in a bowl filled with cold water and swish them around with your hands. Scoop them up and gently blot dry with a paper towel or put them in a salad spinner. Heartier herbs such as rosemary, sage, and marjoram will stay fresh for up to one to two weeks in the refrigerator as long as they remain dry.

When choosing herbs, look for ones with a fresh aroma and avoid those with yellow or limp leaves. Most herbs can be found in bunches, fastened together with a rubber band or twist tie, or in plastic packages in the produce section of most supermarkets.

Ginger: Derived from a rhizome or root, ginger originated in India but is now found throughout Asia. It is light brown in color and has a knotty appearance on the outside but is golden and juicy on the inside. Ginger is both sweet and spicy. Just before using ginger in a recipe, peel away the skin of only the part you are going to use. Store the remaining ginger in a sealed plastic bag in the refrigerator; it will last for several weeks. When buying ginger, choose one with firm knobs and smooth skin. Look for it in the produce section of most supermarkets or in Asian food stores.

Onions and garlic: Like many cooks, I have been accustomed to using onions and garlic liberally in my cooking. I learned that when following a low-carbohydrate diet, however, it is important to be more discerning about the amount and type of onion or garlic included in a recipe. While chives are exceptionally low in carbohydrates, a garlic clove has 1 gram of carbohydrate, ½ cup of chopped leeks has 4 grams, ½ cup of chopped onion has 5, and 1 cup of chopped green onion (or scallion) contains 5 grams of this unwelcome component. If you are not losing weight as quickly as you desire, then it is best to eliminate these ingredients or at least cut in half the amount called for in any recipe.

Useful Information about Kitchen Equipment

It is not essential to have an extensive array of kitchen equipment to be able to prepare low-carbohydrate recipes, but you may find that some of the items discussed here can be useful in helping you achieve the best results with a minimum of effort. Many of these implements are inexpensive. For those that are somewhat more costly, you may find that with a little improvisation some of the equipment you already own can be used for the same purpose:

Blender: A blender consists of a glass, metal, or plastic food container fitted with a metal blade inside at the bottom. It sits on a base with a control panel that allows the blades to spin at different speeds to liquefy, puree, chop, or whip almost any food that is reasonably soft.

Food processor: According to the *New York Times,* the food processor was the "twentieth-century French revolution." This unique appliance comes with special blades and disc attachments that allow it to mince, chop, grate, shred, slice, knead, blend, puree, or liquefy most foods, as well as crush ice. The food processor has a base, directly under the work bowl, that houses the motor. A metal shaft extending from the base through the center of the work bowl connects the blade or disc to the motor. A cover that fits over the work bowl has a feed tube, where you can add ingredients through to the work bowl while the machine is running.

Meat thermometer: A meat thermometer is the most reliable way to determine when food is properly cooked. The thermometer reads the food's internal temperature, which is the true indicator of doneness. You should insert the tip of the thermometer as deep as possible into the item you are testing, but avoid touching the bone. There are many varieties of meat thermometers on the market, but I prefer the instant-read models. Once inserted into the meat, a reading is displayed within seconds. Meat thermometers can be found in most hardware stores or gourmet shops.

Nonreactive cookware: Nonreactive cookware is composed of materials that do not chemically react with certain foods or alter their appearance. Examples of nonreactive materials are ceramic, glass, stainless steel, clay, and plastic. Examples of reactive materials include aluminum, copper, and carbon.

Nonstick cookware: Nonstick cookware is an essential tool for preparing foods if you wish to avoid the addition of fats and oils. A special coating is applied to the cooking surface that allows you to sauté, stir-fry, or fry with little or no fat. This cookware is widely available, and the range of prices makes it affordable for almost any budget.

Parchment paper: The surface of parchment paper is permeable, so it will not soak up moisture and grease. When a harmless silicone coating is applied, it has the added benefit of being a nonstick paper. Another advantage to using parchment paper is that it makes for a faster and easier cleanup—simply discard the paper. It usually comes on rolls, similar to waxed paper and aluminum foil, or in stacks of sheets. You can purchase it in hardware stores, gourmet food shops, and the aluminum foil section of most supermarkets

Pepper mill: A pepper mill is an essential tool for grinding peppercorns. These handy implements, typically made of plastic or wood, come in an assortment of shapes and sizes. Each variety features its own unique mechanism for grinding the peppercorns. Some pepper mills require that you rotate a turnkey or wing nut located on the top, squeeze a handle or bar, or turn a crank handle while for others you must turn the top section, just as you would a doorknob. Another essential feature of a pepper mill is the grinding surface. Be sure to look for one with a machine-cut stainless steel or carbon steel grinding mechanism. Unfortunately, this information is not always apparent. If the pepper mill costs more than $20, however, it is likely that it features this kind of grinding mechanism. Finally, before you buy a pepper mill, be sure to hold it in your hand to determine whether it fits comfortably and is easy to use.

The pepper mill that I prefer, the PepperGun, has spring-loaded handles to squeeze. Although it is designed to be used easily with one hand, I find that I often have to use two hands. Even so, I am always very pleased with the end result. Other pepper mills that get high ratings are the Peugot, Magnum, Peppermate, and Banton, just to name a few. Pepper mills are available in gourmet shops, hardware stores, and department stores, as well as online.

Salad spinner: A salad spinner is one of the easiest ways to dry salad greens and some herbs. You simply place the washed greens in an inner perforated container, then you turn a crank or press down on a knob, which rotates the container rapidly, forcing the water into an outer container that acts as a receptacle. You will find some salad spinners that combine both washing and drying functions. In this variety, you place the greens in a drain basket fitted with a lid that has multiple holes on top. When you set the spinner under cold running water, the soil on the greens is rinsed away. With a few turns of the crank, the leaves are perfectly dry.

Springform pan: A springform is a round pan with high, straight sides that are able to expand with the aid of a spring or clamp. It has a bottom from which the sides of the pan separate when the spring is released. Taking away the sides allows you to remove a cake from the pan without damage to the cake.

Vegetable steamers: I like to use a vegetable steamer whenever possible because it is an excellent way to cook vegetables and still preserve their color, flavor, and vital nutrients. You place the food in a steamer basket or folding colander that sits in a larger covered pot. Boiling water in the bottom of the pot creates steam that cooks the food. If you do not have a vegetable steamer, a footed colander will work equally well.

Wire whisk: Whisks come in a variety of sizes and shapes, each designed to perform a number of different tasks. A *balloon whisk* is often used to add air to a soufflé or meringue or to blend food items in a shallow dish. The *French whisk* is for working with thick sauces or batters while the *standard whisk* is for simple jobs, such as blending dry ingredients.

Cooking Terms Worth Knowing

Creating a low-carbohydrate dish can involve an array of cooking methods. Most are very simple, but it is important to understand the terminology typically used to describe them. I hope you find these brief definitions of some of the terms used throughout this book useful as you begin the creative process of low-carbohydrate cooking:

Blanch: Immerse food briefly in boiling water to set the color or flavor or to make it easier to remove the skin.

Boil: Heat liquid until bubbles appear on the surface.

Broil: Cook food under direct heat provided by a heating element or a hot flame.

Butterfly: Split poultry or meat down the center, cutting almost all the way through, and remove the bone. Fan the poultry or meat open and lay it flat; the resulting shape resembles that of a butterfly.

Chop: Cut food into very fine pieces.

Cube: Cut food into ¼- to ½-inch cubes.

Dice: Cut food into ⅛- to ¼-inch cubes.

Grate: Shred or reduce food into fine particles using a hand grater or a food processor.

Grill: Cook food quickly over high heat.

Julienne: Cut vegetables, meat, or cheese into matchsticks.

Mince: Cut food into cubes of ⅛ inch or less.

Puree: Reduce food to a pastelike consistency, usually by using a food processor or a blender.

Sauté: Cook food quickly in an open pan.

Simmer: Cook food at just below the boiling point.

Steam: Cook food by exposing it to the vapor of boiling liquid.

Stir-fry: Cook food quickly over high heat while constantly stirring.

The pantry is stocked, the refrigerator is full, and you now know how to steam, stir-fry, and dice—so what are you waiting for? I hope you soon discover that following a low-carbohydrate diet can be more satisfying and rewarding than you ever imagined. With such a variety of new, quick, and easy-to-prepare menu choices from which to choose, I am confident that "been there, done that" will quickly disappear from your culinary vocabulary.

A Few Low-Carbohydrate Basics

part two

✦ ✦ ✦ ✦ ✦ ✦ ✦ ✦ ✦

INDULGING

chapter four

APPETIZER
EXCITEMENT

APPETIZERS

A-B-C Dip

Cheddar Cheese Balls

Cheese Crisps

Chicken Terrine

Chinese Chicken Wings

Chinese Pork and Shrimp
    Stuffed Mushrooms

Chinese Shrimp Kebabs

Clam Dip

Creamy Herb Dip

Curry Dip

Deviled Eggs

Eggplant and Red Pepper Dip

Greek Yogurt and Cucumber
    Dip (Tsatziki)

Guacamole

Hot Artichoke Dip

Hot Crab Dip

Hot and Spicy Pecans

Italian Tuna and Cheese
    Spread

Liptauer Cheese Spread

Marinated Artichokes and
    Mushrooms

Marinated Asparagus

Maytag Blue Cheese Dip

Mushrooms Stuffed with
    Italian Sausage

Pine Nut Dip

Red Salmon Mousse

Roasted Red Pepper Dip

Smoked Salmon Mousse

Smoked Salmon Pinwheels

Smoked Trout Mousse on
    Cucumber Rounds

Tapenade

WHETHER YOU ARE HOSTING an intimate dinner, sharing the holiday season with loved ones, or gathered around the television with friends, nothing is more welcoming than a tray laden with an assortment of appealing appetizers. Imagine a tasty array such as a savory cheese ball, a zesty vegetable dip, and a few finger foods. Fortunately, these delights are among the easiest low-carbohydrate foods to prepare and enjoy. Often, they are made with such ingredients as cheese, bacon, mayonnaise, seafood, or nuts. Although low in carbohydrates, these morsels are bursting with an impressive range of temptingly delicious flavors. What's even better, the majority of these bite-size gems can be made ahead so you are free to do other things when guests arrive.

Not only are appetizers a wonderful food to share with family and friends, they also can stave off hunger in an emergency. Some diets even recommend a snack between meals, but the regimen you have chosen determines the kind and amount you can indulge in. Of course, as with all good things, moderation is suggested. As many of these delightful savories are made with rich ingredients, you may want to save your healthiest appetite for the salad, low-carbohydrate vegetables, and meat portions of your meal that follows. Also, please note that although I have included ingredients that are not reduced fat, such substitutions are always in order. In most instances, the flavor and texture are not significantly compromised by a low-fat substitution while the calorie count and fat grams can be greatly reduced. For those recipes where substitutions are not advisable, I have made a notation to that effect.

So, fill your platter with an assortment of celery sticks, zucchini spears, and cauliflower florets, spread out some low-carbohydrate crackers with a bowl of Creamy Herb Dip in the center, and let the party begin.

A-B-C Dip

This dip is as easy to prepare as A-B-C. It is also simply delicious! Serve with an assortment of low-carbohydrate vegetables
or crackers.

8 TO 10 SERVINGS

1½ cups grated sharp Cheddar
   cheese
¾ cup mayonnaise
⅓ cup slivered almonds,
   toasted*

3 strips bacon, cooked, drained,
   and crumbled
1 tablespoon finely minced
   yellow onion
¼ teaspoon coarse salt

COMBINE all ingredients in a medium bowl and mix lightly. Refrigerate, covered, for up to 4 hours. Bring to room temperature before serving.

EACH SERVING PROVIDES:
1g carbohydrates, 279 calories, 7g protein, 27g fat,
0g dietary fiber, 399mg sodium, 42mg cholesterol

*To toast the almonds: Preheat oven to 350 degrees F. Place the almonds in a shallow
pan and bake for 10 to 15 minutes or until golden brown.

Cheddar Cheese Balls

For large parties, I often make this recipe into one large ball, coat it with finely chopped pecans, and serve it alongside an assortment of crackers. The mixture is thick enough to form into small balls instead, making it attractive to low-carbohydrate dieters. By inserting toothpicks into each one, these savories become a delicious treat to be enjoyed sans carbohydrate-laden crackers.

10 TO 12 CHEESE BALLS

1 pound grated sharp Cheddar cheese, at room temperature

1 package (8 ounces) cream cheese, at room temperature

1 to 1¼ ounces Maytag Blue Cheese or favorite blue cheese, at room temperature

1 teaspoon minced yellow onion

1 teaspoon Worcestershire sauce

½ cup dried parsley flakes

Garlic salt to taste

COMBINE all ingredients in the work bowl of a food processor fitted with a metal blade (or in an electric mixer or blender) and process until well blended. Transfer the mixture to a covered dish and refrigerate for 1 to 2 hours or until firm. Pinch off 1 tablespoon and roll it between the palm of your hands to form a round ball. Repeat this process with the remaining cheese mixture.

VARIATION: Roll the cheese balls in finely chopped pecans.

EACH SERVING PROVIDES:
2g carbohydrates, 276 calories, 14g protein, 24g fat,
0g dietary fiber, 398mg sodium, 75mg cholesterol

Cheese Crisps

Cheese crisps, sometimes referred to as fricos, provide just the right amount of satisfaction when you are looking for something delicious and crispy to munch on. They can be served as an appetizer, as an accompaniment to soup or salad, or even used to scoop up a creamy dip. To make perfect cheese crisps, grate the cheese just before you are ready to prepare them. This will prevent any loss of moisture and assure even melting and more perfectly shaped crisps.

10 CHEESE CRISPS

1 teaspoon cumin seeds*
2 cups freshly grated sharp
   Cheddar cheese**

PREHEAT oven to 425 degrees F. Line a baking sheet with parchment paper. Set aside. Place a small pan over medium heat for 2 minutes. Add the cumin seeds and toast for 3 to 4 minutes or until the seeds become fragrant, stirring occasionally. Remove the pan from the heat and allow the seeds to cool for 5 minutes. Transfer the cumin seeds to a spice grinder and grind into a powder.

Combine the freshly grated cheese and cumin powder in a large bowl and blend well. On one-quarter of the prepared baking sheet, sprinkle about 2 tablespoons of the cheese to form a circle about 4 inches in diameter. Repeat with three more circles. Bake for 5 to 6 minutes or just until the cheese begins to show some color. Do not let the cheese get too dark because it will taste bitter and lose its delicate

---

*Instead of the cumin seeds, ¾ teaspoon ground cumin can be used. In that case, simply mix the powder with the cheese.

**Do not substitute reduced-fat or nonfat Cheddar cheese in this recipe.

cheese flavor. Remove the pan from the oven and place it on a cake rack. Allow the cheese crisps to cool for about 5 minutes or until you can slide a spatula under the edges and lift them off the sheet. Transfer them to a double thickness of paper towels and cool completely.

EACH SERVING PROVIDES:

0g carbohydrates, 92 calories, 6g protein, 8g fat,

0g dietary fiber, 141mg sodium, 24mg cholesterol

Chicken Terrine

If you are daunted at the thought of making a terrine, you will be pleasantly surprised to experience how easy it is to prepare this treat. Just make sure to have all the ingredients nearby, and you are ready to go. Best of all, it can be prepared a day ahead. This terrine can be served as a first course or even enjoyed as a luncheon main course.

8 SERVINGS

1 pound pork sausage, casing removed
2 tablespoons butter (or extra virgin olive oil)
½ cup chopped yellow onion
½ teaspoon dried thyme leaves
¼ teaspoon dried tarragon leaves
2 eggs, slightly beaten
3 tablespoons cognac or brandy

3 tablespoons chopped fresh parsley
½ teaspoon coarse salt
¼ teaspoon freshly ground pepper
1 pound skinless and boneless chicken breast halves, each cut in half lengthwise
10 slices bacon

PREHEAT oven to 400 degrees F. Coarsely chop the pork sausage. Heat the butter in a large skillet over medium heat. Add the onion and sauté for 5 minutes or until golden brown, stirring occasionally. Add the thyme, tarragon, and sausage and blend well. Cook for another 5 minutes or until the sausage is brown, stirring frequently. Remove the skillet from the heat, add the eggs, cognac, parsley, salt, and pepper, and blend well.

Place the chicken breasts between sheets of waxed paper. Pound them with a mallet to flatten them to ¼ to ½ inch.

Line a 9 × 5-inch loaf pan with 6 slices of bacon. Make alternate layers of the chicken and sausage mixture, beginning and ending with the chicken. It is okay if the layers are not even. Place the remaining 4 slices of bacon on top of the chicken and tuck the bacon ends into the pan. Bake for 1 hour.

Before serving the terrine, drain the fat. Cut the terrine into 8 slices and serve warm or cold. Garnish each serving with a sprig of parsley, if desired.

EACH SERVING PROVIDES:

2g carbohydrates, 397 calories, 32g protein, 27g fat,
0g dietary fiber, 931mg sodium, 147mg cholesterol

Chinese Chicken Wings

These richly flavored chicken wings are certain to become a favorite. Who would believe anything this good could be so low in carbohydrates!

4 SERVINGS

2 tablespoons oyster sauce
2 tablespoons cold water
1½ tablespoons soy sauce
1½ tablespoons Asian sesame oil
1 tablespoon medium dry
   sherry
1 piece fresh ginger, cut 1-inch
   thick and minced

1 clove garlic, minced
1 teaspoon Splenda or other
   artificial sweetener
½ teaspoon coarse salt
2 pounds (or 8) chicken wings,
   wing tips removed

PREHEAT oven to 375 degrees F. Line a baking sheet with aluminum foil. Set aside.

In a large resealable plastic bag, combine all the ingredients except the chicken wings, and blend to make marinade.

Cut each chicken wing into two pieces. Add the chicken wings to the marinade and turn to coat all over. Seal the bag and refrigerate for 1 hour or more, turning the chicken pieces occasionally.

Lightly coat the lined baking sheet with a nonstick vegetable spray. Remove the chicken wings from the marinade (discard the marinade) and place them on the baking sheet. Bake for 1 hour, turning the chicken wings every 15 minutes to ensure they brown evenly.

EACH SERVING PROVIDES:
0g carbohydrates, 267 calories, 24g protein, 18g fat,
0g dietary fiber, 273mg sodium, 73mg cholesterol

Chinese Pork and Shrimp Stuffed Mushrooms

These stuffed mushrooms are sensational! The filling can be made early in the day and stuffed in the mushrooms a few hours before you are ready to serve them.

24 STUFFED MUSHROOMS

24 large mushrooms, stems removed
¼ cup extra virgin olive oil
Coarse salt for sprinkling, plus 1 teaspoon
½ pound ground pork
¼ pound cooked shrimp, peeled, deveined, and finely chopped

3 tablespoons chopped green onion
1 tablespoon soy sauce
¼ teaspoon freshly ground pepper

PREHEAT oven to 425 degrees F. Place the mushrooms in a large re-sealable plastic bag and add the olive oil. Seal the bag and turn the mushrooms to coat all over.

Place the mushrooms, stem side up, on a rimmed baking sheet. Sprinkle a little salt inside each cap. Bake the mushrooms in the oven for 10 minutes. Turn the mushrooms over and bake for another 6 minutes. Place the mushrooms, stem side down, on a double thickness of paper towels. Set aside for about 10 minutes. (Although the mushrooms can be stuffed without first baking them, this method assures they will not be soggy or drip. Preparing mushrooms this way not only extracts any excess moisture but it also enhances their flavor.)

(continues)

Reduce oven heat to 400 degrees F. Combine the pork, shrimp, green onion, soy sauce, salt, and pepper in a small bowl and blend well. Stuff the mushrooms with the filling, dividing evenly. Bake for 20 to 25 minutes or until the filling is firm to the touch.

EACH SERVING PROVIDES:

1g carbohydrates, 40 calories, 3g protein, 3g fat,

0g dietary fiber, 134mg sodium, 12mg cholesterol

Chinese Shrimp Kebabs

You will find any excuse to make these spicy appetizers. Left-over shrimp can be used in the Shrimp and Mushroom Salad (page 132).

4 KEBABS

¼ cup soy sauce

2 tablespoons chopped garlic

2 tablespoons chopped fresh ginger

2 tablespoons thinly sliced green onion

2 tablespoons Splenda or other artificial sweetener

1 teaspoon Asian sesame oil

¼ teaspoon dried red pepper flakes

1½ pounds medium raw shrimp, peeled and deveined

IN a medium resealable plastic bag, combine all the ingredients except the shrimp and blend well to make the marinade. Add the shrimp and turn to coat all over. Seal the bag and refrigerate for 4 to 5 hours, turning the shrimp occasionally.

Preheat the broiler. Remove the shrimp from the marinade and thread them onto 8-inch wooden skewers that have soaked in water for at least 30 minutes. Set a rack over a broiler-proof pan and place the shrimp on the rack. Place the pan under the broiler, 3 inches from the heat source, and broil the shrimp for 3 to 4 minutes on each side or until they are pink.

VARIATION: Place the shrimp on a baking sheet that has been lightly coated with a nonstick vegetable spray and bake in a preheated oven at 400 degrees F for 10 to 12 minutes.

EACH SERVING PROVIDES:
7g carbohydrates, 218 calories, 36g protein, 4g fat,
0g dietary fiber, 1215mg sodium, 259mg cholesterol

Clam Dip

Most of the ingredients found in this easy-to-prepare Clam Dip can be stored in your refrigerator and pantry to have on hand when you need to whip up a snack for unexpected guests.

6 TO 8 SERVINGS

1 package (8 ounces) cream cheese, at room temperature
1 teaspoon minced fresh parsley
¾ teaspoon garlic powder
¼ teaspoon coarse salt
¼ teaspoon Worcestershire sauce

1 to 2 drops (or more) Tabasco sauce or other hot pepper sauce
1 can (10 ounces) minced clams, drained

COMBINE all the ingredients except the clams in a medium bowl and blend until smooth. Add the clams and blend well. The clam dip can be served immediately or kept in a covered dish in the refrigerator for several hours or overnight. Bring to room temperature before serving. Serve with an assortment of low-carbohydrate veggies or crackers.

EACH SERVING PROVIDES:
3g carbohydrates, 153 calories, 6g protein, 13g fat,
0g dietary fiber, 390mg sodium, 49mg cholesterol

Creamy Herb Dip

This dip is easy to make but difficult to keep from eating all at one sitting. Serve with an assortment of low-carbohydrate veggies.

6 SERVINGS

2 cloves garlic

2 tablespoons fresh lemon juice

1 egg*

½ cup freshly grated Parmesan cheese

½ cup chopped fresh parsley

1 teaspoon dried basil

½ teaspoon coarse salt

⅛ teaspoon (or less) cayenne pepper

½ cup extra virgin olive oil

½ cup plain yogurt

PLACE the garlic in the work bowl of a food processor fitted with a metal blade (or in a blender) and process until finely chopped. Add the lemon juice, egg, cheese, parsley, basil, salt, and cayenne and process until smooth. With the motor running, add the olive oil in a slow, steady stream and process until the mixture is thick and well blended. Add the yogurt and lightly blend. Transfer the dip to a covered container and refrigerate for several hours or overnight.

EACH SERVING PROVIDES:

3g carbohydrates, 236 calories, 5g protein, 23g fat,
0g dietary fiber, 334mg sodium, 40mg cholesterol

*If you are concerned about adding a raw egg to the dip, simply omit the egg. The dip may not be quite as thick, but it will still be delicious.

Curry Dip

You will find yourself dreaming up novel ways to serve this dip other than as a snack. As a suggestion, it would make a delightful sauce spooned over grilled tuna or salmon or even served to adorn steamed broccoli or asparagus.

8 SERVINGS

1 cup mayonnaise
½ cup sour cream
1 tablespoon minced yellow
   onion
1 tablespoon minced fresh
   parsley

1½ teaspoons fresh lemon juice
1 to 2 teaspoons curry powder
1 teaspoon Fines Herbs
½ teaspoon Worcestershire
   sauce
¼ teaspoon coarse salt

COMBINE all ingredients in a medium bowl and mix well. Cover the bowl and refrigerate for several hours or overnight to allow the flavors to blend.

EACH SERVING PROVIDES:

1g carbohydrates, 232 calories, 1g protein, 25g fat,
0g dietary fiber, 220mg sodium, 33mg cholesterol

Deviled Eggs

Deviled eggs are the perfect treat to indulge in when you are watching your carbohydrates. They are delicately spiced and satisfying at the same time. When piped into egg white halves and garnished with a sprig of parsley, these devilish treats become an elegant addition to serve at a cocktail party.

7 SERVINGS

14 large eggs
6 tablespoons mayonnaise
½ tablespoon grainy mustard
1 tablespoon cider vinegar or favorite vinegar
½ teaspoon Worcestershire sauce

½ teaspoon coarse salt
½ teaspoon freshly ground pepper
1 to 2 dashes of Tabasco sauce or favorite hot pepper sauce (optional)

PLACE the eggs in a large saucepan filled with enough water to come 1 inch above the eggs. Place the saucepan over high heat and bring to a rolling boil. Once the water comes to a boil, turn off the heat, cover, and leave the saucepan on the burner for 30 minutes or until the water is tepid. Remove the eggs from the water. Crack each egg all over and hold it under cold running water while removing the shell. Place the eggs on a double thickness of paper towels to dry. Put the eggs in a covered container and refrigerate until needed.

To prepare the deviled eggs, slice each egg in half lengthwise with a sharp knife. Carefully remove the egg yolks (reserve the egg whites) and put them in a medium bowl. Mash the egg yolks with a fork into a smooth paste. Add the rest of the ingredients and blend well. Taste for seasoning. Spoon the yolk mixture into the egg white halves, dividing evenly. (There may not be enough filling to fill all of the egg white halves.) For a decorative touch, instead of spooning the filling

(continues)

into the eggs, spoon it into a pastry bag (or you can use a freezer bag by cutting one of the corners) fitted with a ½-inch star tip and pipe it into the egg white halves so it slightly mounds. Lightly sprinkle the tops with paprika and garnish each with a sprig of parsley.

VARIATION: To make curried deviled eggs, follow the instructions in the above recipe except combine the mashed egg yolks with ½ cup mayonnaise, 2 tablespoons minced green onion, and 1½ teaspoons curry powder (omit the other ingredients).

EACH SERVING PROVIDES:

2g carbohydrates, 276 calories, 15g protein, 23g fat,
0g dietary fiber, 400mg sodium, 506mg cholesterol

Eggplant and Red Pepper Dip

When choosing an eggplant, look for one that has a round blossom end rather than an oval one. The male eggplant has the round blossom end and its seeds are less bitter than the female variety.

4 SERVINGS

1 red bell pepper
1 (1 pound) eggplant
4 tablespoons extra virgin
   olive oil
2 cloves garlic
2 tablespoons tahini*
1 tablespoon plain yogurt

1 teaspoon ground cumin
½ teaspoon coarse salt
¼ teaspoon freshly ground
   pepper
2 tablespoons chopped fresh
   parsley

PREHEAT the broiler. Place the red pepper on a baking sheet lined with aluminum foil. Broil the pepper, turning it as the skin blackens, for 20 minutes or until the skin is charred all over. Once the pepper is roasted, place it in a plastic bag, seal, and allow it to steam for 15 to 20 minutes. When the pepper is cool enough to handle, peel away the skin and remove the top and seeds. (Do not rinse the pepper.) Set aside.

Preheat oven to 400 degrees F. While the red pepper is cooling, peel the eggplant and cut into 1-inch cubes. Place the cubes in a resealable plastic bag and add 3 tablespoons olive oil. Seal the bag and roll the cubes in the oil to coat them all over. Place the cubes on a baking pan that has been lightly sprayed with a nonstick vegetable spray. Bake for 45 minutes or until the eggplant is fork tender and brown. Cool slightly.

(continues)

*Tahini is made of toasted and hulled sesame seeds that are ground into a paste. It is available in most health food stores or Middle-Eastern food stores.

Place the garlic in the work bowl of a food processor fitted with a metal blade (or in a blender) and process until chopped. Add the eggplant and red pepper and finely chop. Add the tahini, 1 tablespoon olive oil, yogurt, cumin, salt, and pepper and process until blended. Add the parsley and pulse to blend. Transfer the eggplant and red pepper dip to a covered container and refrigerate for several hours or overnight.

EACH SERVING PROVIDES:
12g carbohydrates, 171 calories, 3g protein, 14g fat,
4g dietary fiber, 245mg sodium, 0mg cholesterol

Greek Yogurt and Cucumber Dip (Tsatziki)

You will enjoy serving this cooling dip with an assortment of low-carbohydrate vegetables on a hot and sultry summer day. The dip is equally as delicious when it is used as a condiment to enhance the flavors of many of the Mediterranean recipes found throughout this book, especially Greek Chicken (page 197) or Mediterranean Turkey Patties (page 229).

8 SERVINGS

1 English (hothouse or seedless) cucumber, cut into julienne strips (or 2 small cucumbers, peeled and cut into julienne strips)

1 tablespoon coarse salt

¾ cup plain nonfat yogurt

¾ cup sour cream*

3 tablespoons extra virgin olive oil

4 cloves garlic, minced

1½ tablespoons chopped fresh dill (or 1 to 2 teaspoons dried dill weed)

1½ tablespoons fresh lemon juice

¼ teaspoon freshly ground pepper

SET a strainer over a bowl. Place the cucumber in the strainer and sprinkle with the salt. Allow the cucumber to sit for 1 hour. Rinse. Pat dry with paper towels. Combine the cucumber and the rest of the ingredients in a medium bowl and blend well. The dip should be served soon after it is prepared, otherwise it tends to get watery. Stir before serving and taste for seasoning.

EACH SERVING PROVIDES:

4g carbohydrates, 112 calories, 2g protein, 9g fat,

0g dietary fiber, 736mg sodium, 19mg cholesterol

*Do not substitute reduced-fat sour cream in this recipe.

Guacamole

A good friend gave this guacamole recipe to me and I have been using it ever since. I like to serve it as a dip with low-carbohydrate veggies or to enhance a fajita salad—let your imagination guide you to find other ways to serve this zesty dip.

8 SERVINGS

2 ripe avocados, peeled
2 tablespoons salsa
2 tablespoons fresh lemon juice
2 teaspoons mayonnaise

⅛ teaspoon garlic powder
⅛ teaspoon coarse salt
⅛ teaspoon cayenne pepper

PLACE the avocado pulp (reserve one pit) in a small bowl and mash with a fork until smooth. Add the rest of the ingredients and blend well. If not serving the guacamole immediately, place the reserved pit in the center of the dip to prevent it from turning brown. Cover the bowl with plastic wrap and refrigerate. Or, omit the avocado pit and place the plastic wrap directly on top of the dip so it is sealed airtight.

EACH SERVING PROVIDES:
4g carbohydrates, 92 calories, 1g protein, 9g fat,
3g dietary fiber, 58mg sodium, 1mg cholesterol

Hot Artichoke Dip

This sensational dip is so easy to prepare yet decadently delicious and low in carbohydrates. Serve with an assortment of low-carb vegetables or crackers.

8 TO 10 SERVINGS

1 cup mayonnaise

1 can (14 ounces) artichoke hearts, drained and chopped

1 cup freshly grated Parmesan cheese

¼ teaspoon seasoned salt

PREHEAT the oven to 350 degrees F. Combine all ingredients in a small bowl and blend well. Transfer the dip to a 2-cup ovenproof dish and bake for 30 minutes.

EACH SERVING PROVIDES:

4g carbohydrates, 278 calories, 6g protein, 26g fat,

1g dietary fiber, 571mg sodium, 30mg cholesterol

Hot Crab Dip

This make-ahead crab dip is the perfect reward for following a low-carbohydrate diet. Throw away the rich crackers and enjoy this creamy dip with an assortment of veggie sticks or low-carb crackers.

12 SERVINGS

1 can (6 to 8 ounces) lump crabmeat, drained and flaked

1 package (8 ounces) cream cheese, at room temperature

½ cup mayonnaise

1 tablespoon chopped fresh chives

¼ teaspoon Tabasco sauce or other hot pepper sauce

½ teaspoon Worcestershire sauce

PLACE all ingredients in the work bowl of a food processor fitted with a metal blade (or in a mixer or blender) and process until smooth. Spoon the crab dip into a 1-quart ceramic or glass dish. Microwave on high power for 90 seconds (or bake in an oven at 300 degrees F for 25 to 30 minutes) or until it is hot and bubbly. (The dip can also be made one day ahead. Transfer it to a covered dish and refrigerate until ready to heat in microwave or oven.)

EACH SERVING PROVIDES:
1g carbohydrates, 147 calories, 4g protein, 14g fat,
0g dietary fiber, 156mg sodium, 40mg cholesterol

Hot and Spicy Pecans

These hot and spicy pecans are the ideal snack to serve when having friends over for a casual meal. I must warn you, however—they can be addictive!

8 SERVINGS

¼ cup canola oil
¼ cup Worcestershire sauce
½ teaspoon seasoned salt

8 to 10 dashes Tabasco sauce or
favorite hot pepper sauce
1 pound pecans

PREHEAT oven to 300 degrees F. Line a baking sheet with aluminum foil. Set aside.

Combine the oil, Worcestershire sauce, seasoned salt, and hot pepper sauce in a large bowl and blend well. Add the pecans and stir until they are completely coated with the oil mixture. Spread the pecans in a single layer on the prepared baking sheet. Bake for 30 minutes, turning the pecans after 15 minutes. Allow the pecans to cool before storing in airtight container.

EACH SERVING PROVIDES:
12g carbohydrates, 447 calories, 5g protein, 45g fat,
4g dietary fiber, 157mg sodium, 0mg cholesterol

Italian Tuna and Cheese Spread

This is a fabulously delicious spread that can be made into small balls and served on toothpicks, piped onto cucumber rounds, or served as a dip with assorted vegetables. Just make sure you choose a sweet Gorgonzola cheese because the other kind has a very pungent aroma and taste.

12 SERVINGS

2 packages (8 ounces each) cream cheese, at room temperature

1/4 pound Dulce (sweet) Gorgonzola cheese, at room temperature*

2 tablespoons minced fresh chives

1 cup pine nuts or chopped walnuts

1 can (7 ounces) tuna with oil

1/2 teaspoon freshly ground pepper

1/4 teaspoon cayenne pepper

2 tablespoons minced fresh parsley

PLACE all ingredients except for the parsley in the work bowl of a food processor fitted with a metal blade (or in a blender) and process until smooth. Add the parsley and pulse to blend lightly. Transfer the spread to a covered dish and refrigerate for several hours or overnight.

EACH SERVING PROVIDES:

3g carbohydrates, 253 calories, 13g protein, 22g fat,

1g dietary fiber, 275mg sodium, 58mg cholesterol

*Blue cheese can be substituted for the Gorgonzola cheese.

Liptauer Cheese Spread

Liptauer cheese spread is of Hungarian origin. It is composed of a combination of unique ingredients that richly contribute to the cheese's memorable flavor.

8 SERVINGS

6 ounces cream cheese, at room temperature
2 ounces (4 tablespoons) butter, at room temperature
2 anchovies, drained and finely chopped
1 finely chopped shallot

1 teaspoon chopped capers
1 teaspoon paprika
$\frac{1}{2}$ teaspoon caraway seeds
$\frac{1}{2}$ teaspoon coarse salt
$\frac{1}{4}$ teaspoon freshly ground pepper

PLACE the cream cheese and butter in a medium bowl and mix until smooth. Add the rest of the ingredients and blend well. Place the spread in a covered bowl or form into a roll and wrap in plastic wrap. Refrigerate for several hours or overnight to allow the spread to season.

EACH SERVING PROVIDES:

4g carbohydrates, 118 calories, 3g protein, 10g fat,
0g dietary fiber, 233mg sodium, 32mg cholesterol

Marinated Artichokes and Mushrooms

Marinated vegetables can be served at parties, as part of a salad course, or when you feel hungry for a quick, healthy snack. For parties, I usually double and triple the recipe and add cauliflower florets or some steamed baby carrots for nondieters.

8 SERVINGS

½ cup extra virgin olive oil
¼ cup tarragon vinegar
3 tablespoons cold water
2 cloves garlic, minced
1 teaspoon dried oregano leaves
1 teaspoon dried basil
1½ teaspoons coarse salt
¼ teaspoon freshly ground pepper

¼ teaspoon Accent (optional)
4 jars (4 ounces each) button mushrooms, drained
2 cans (14 ounces each) artichoke hearts, drained (or 2 packages frozen artichoke hearts, cooked and drained)

IN a jar with a tight-fitting lid, combine all the ingredients except the mushrooms and artichokes and shake well to make the marinade. Place the mushrooms and artichokes in a large jar that has a lid, add the marinade, and blend well. Cover the jar and refrigerate for one week, turning the vegetables each day.

EACH SERVING PROVIDES:
10g carbohydrates, 174 calories, 4g protein, 14g fat,
2g dietary fiber, 827mg sodium, 0mg cholesterol

Marinated Asparagus

Asparagus comes alive when immersed in this delicious Asian-inspired marinade. Halved asparagus can be enjoyed as a snack or the whole spears are delicious served on a bed of greens as a salad.

4 TO 6 SERVINGS

1 pound asparagus spears,
   tough ends removed
2 tablespoons Asian sesame oil

2 tablespoons soy sauce
1 clove garlic, minced

FILL a large bowl with ice water and set aside. Bring water to a rolling boil in a large skillet. Add the asparagus and blanch for 1 minute. Transfer the asparagus to a colander to drain quickly, then immediately immerse it in the ice water. Drain. Pat dry with paper towels.

Combine the sesame oil, soy sauce, and garlic in a dish large enough to hold the asparagus in one layer and blend well. Add the asparagus and turn to coat all over. Cover the dish and refrigerate for up to 4 days, turning the asparagus occasionally.

EACH SERVING PROVIDES:

6g carbohydrates, 94 calories, 3g protein, 7g fat,
2g dietary fiber, 517mg sodium, 0mg cholesterol

Maytag Blue Cheese Dip

This blue cheese dip is certain to satisfy your taste buds. It features world-famous Maytag Blue Cheese, which is produced in Newton, Iowa, and is acclaimed by food experts as the finest American blue cheese. And yes, the same family that makes washing machines created this cheese. Serve this delectable dip with steamed broccoli or low-carbohydrate crackers. For a different taste sensation, spoon some of this delightful dip over hamburgers.

8 SERVINGS

1 cup mayonnaise
½ cup Maytag Blue Cheese
   or favorite blue cheese,
   crumbled

¼ cup sour cream
2 tablespoons fresh lemon juice
1 teaspoon Worcestershire sauce

COMBINE all ingredients in a medium bowl and blend well. Refrigerate, covered, for several hours or overnight.

EACH SERVING PROVIDES:
1g carbohydrates, 246 calories, 2g protein, 26g fat,
0g dietary fiber, 277mg sodium, 33mg cholesterol

Mushrooms Stuffed with Italian Sausage

For easier preparation, the mushrooms do not have to be baked before stuffing them with the Italian sausage. I have found, however, that by baking the mushrooms first, you avoid ones that are soggy and tend to drip. Preparing mushrooms this way not only extracts excess moisture but also enhances their flavor.

24 STUFFED MUSHROOMS

24 large mushrooms, stems removed
¼ cup extra virgin olive oil
Coarse salt
12 ounces sweet or hot Italian sausage

6 to 8 tablespoons freshly grated Parmesan cheese
Dried oregano leaves

PREHEAT oven to 425 degrees F. Place the mushrooms in a large resealable plastic bag and add the olive oil. Seal the bag and turn the mushrooms to coat all over.

Place the mushrooms, stem side up, on a rimmed baking sheet. Sprinkle a little salt inside each cap. Bake the mushrooms for 10 minutes. Turn the mushrooms over and bake for another 6 minutes. Place the mushrooms, stem side down, on a double thickness of paper towels. Set aside for about 10 minutes.

Reduce oven heat to 350 degrees F. Stuff the mushrooms with the sausage and sprinkle the tops with a generous amount of Parmesan cheese and a touch of oregano. Bake for 20 minutes.

EACH SERVING PROVIDES:
1g carbohydrates, 80 calories, 4g protein, 7g fat,
0g dietary fiber, 161mg sodium, 12mg cholesterol

Pine Nut Dip

You will adore this savory Mediterranean dip. It is sensational spooned over Spicy Chicken Thighs (page 256) or is equally delectable when served as a dip with endive leaves or your favorite low-carbohydrate vegetables.

12 SERVINGS

1 cup pine nuts
2 cloves garlic
5 tablespoons tahini*
2 tablespoons plain yogurt
¼ cup fresh lemon juice
¼ cup (or more) cold water
1 tablespoon extra virgin
   olive oil

½ teaspoon coarse salt
¼ teaspoon freshly ground
   pepper
⅛ teaspoon cayenne pepper
¼ cup minced fresh cilantro or
   parsley

PLACE the pine nuts and garlic in the work bowl of a food processor fitted with a metal blade (or in a blender) and process until the mixture forms a paste. Add the tahini, yogurt, and lemon juice and blend well. Add the water, one tablespoon at a time, and process until the dip is the consistency of sour cream. Add the olive oil, salt, pepper, and cayenne and blend. Add the cilantro or parsley and pulse to blend lightly. Taste for seasoning. If serving the sauce as a dip, garnish the top with a sprig of parsley or cilantro.

EACH SERVING PROVIDES:
3g carbohydrates, 117 calories, 4g protein, 11g fat,
1g dietary fiber, 82mg sodium, 0mg cholesterol

*Tahini is made of toasted and hulled sesame seeds that are ground into a paste. It is available in most health food stores or Middle-Eastern food stores.

Red Salmon Mousse

Red salmon is a great component for an appetizer mousse because it is densely flavored and richly colored. Serve this delicacy in a dish and place it alongside a basket of low-carbohydrate crackers. Or, to gussy it up, pipe or spread the mousse onto 1/4-inch-thick English cucumber rounds or ends of endive leaves and garnish each with a sprig of fresh dill or parsley.

8 TO 10 SERVINGS

1/3 cup fresh parsley
1 can (14 ounces) red salmon, drained, bones and skin removed
3 tablespoons chopped green onion, green part only
2 tablespoons fresh lemon juice

2 tablespoons mayonnaise
1 tablespoon whipping cream
1 tablespoon Dijon mustard
1/2 teaspoon coarse salt
1/2 teaspoon freshly ground pepper

PLACE the parsley in the work bowl of a food processor fitted with a metal blade (or in a blender) and process until finely chopped. Add the rest of the ingredients and process just until smooth. Transfer the red salmon mousse to a serving dish, cover, and refrigerate for several hours or overnight.

EACH SERVING PROVIDES:
1g carbohydrates, 123 calories, 11g protein, 9g fat,
0g dietary fiber, 399mg sodium, 37mg cholesterol

Roasted Red Pepper Dip

One taste of this decadently rich dip and you will want to make it over and over again. This delicious dip, served with an assortment of vegetables, can be made a day ahead. Just remember to bring it to room temperature before serving.

12 SERVINGS

2 red bell peppers
8 green onions, white part only
¼ cup fresh cilantro leaves
2 cloves garlic
⅓ cup chopped sun-dried tomatoes in olive oil, drained

1 package (8 ounces) cream
cheese, at room temperature
2 teaspoons ground cumin
¼ teaspoon coarse salt

To roast the red peppers, place them on a baking sheet lined with aluminum foil and broil them under a preheated broiler. Broil for 20 minutes or until the skins are charred all over, turning the peppers as the skin blackens. After roasting, place the peppers in a plastic bag, seal, and allow them to steam for 15 to 20 minutes. When the peppers are cool enough to handle, peel away the skin and remove the top and seeds. (Do not rinse the peppers.)

Place the green onions, cilantro, and garlic in the work bowl of a food processor fitted with a metal blade (or in a blender) and process until finely chopped. Add the roasted red peppers and sun-dried tomatoes and process just until blended. Add the cream cheese, cumin, and salt and blend well. Transfer the roasted red pepper dip to a serving dish. The dip can be served immediately or refrigerated, covered, for several hours or overnight.

EACH SERVING PROVIDES:
3g carbohydrates, 81 calories, 2g protein, 7g fat,
1g dietary fiber, 105mg sodium, 21mg cholesterol

Smoked Salmon Mousse

The smoky flavor of smoked salmon transforms this delicious mousse into a memorable treat. It can be served in a dish alongside vegetables or low-carbohydrate crackers or decoratively piped into celery sticks or onto $\frac{1}{4}$-inch-thick cucumber rounds and garnished with a bit of parsley or dill.

8 SERVINGS

1 package (4.5 ounces) smoked salmon, broken into small pieces, skin removed

1 tablespoon fresh lemon juice

6 tablespoons melted butter

$\frac{1}{2}$ cup sour cream

1 tablespoon chopped fresh dill (or $\frac{1}{2}$ teaspoon dried dill weed)

$\frac{1}{4}$ teaspoon coarse salt

$\frac{1}{4}$ teaspoon freshly ground pepper

PLACE the salmon and lemon juice in the work bowl of a food processor fitted with a metal blade (or in a blender) and process until finely chopped. Add the butter in a slow, steady stream and blend until smooth. Add the rest of the ingredients and blend until smooth. Transfer the mousse to a dish, cover, and refrigerate for several hours or overnight. Bring to room temperature before serving.

VARIATION: To top cucumber rounds with smoked salmon mousse, cut an English (hothouse or seedless) cucumber into $\frac{1}{4}$-inch-thick slices. Spoon the smoked salmon mousse into a pastry bag (or you can use a freezer bag by cutting one of the corners) fitted with a $\frac{1}{2}$-inch star tip. Pipe rosettes in the center of each cucumber round and garnish with a small piece of fresh dill or parsley. The cucumber rounds can be prepared 4 hours ahead. Place them in a rimmed pan that is higher than the rosettes, cover with plastic wrap, and refrigerate.

EACH SERVING PROVIDES:
1g carbohydrates, 126 calories, 4g protein, 12g fat,
0g dietary fiber, 193mg sodium, 39mg cholesterol

Smoked Salmon Pinwheels

Lox and cream cheese are a classic breakfast combination. You will be especially pleased to find how easy it is to prepare these bite-size gems and how delicious they are to eat.

6 SERVINGS

4 ounces cream cheese, at room temperature

2 tablespoons minced fresh chives

1 tablespoon minced fresh dill (or 1 teaspoon dried dill weed)

2 teaspoons capers, rinsed and drained

⅛ teaspoon freshly ground pepper

6 ounces thinly sliced smoked salmon (lox)

COMBINE the cream cheese, chives, dill, capers, and pepper in a small bowl and mix until well blended.

Place a slice of smoked salmon on a work surface and spread a thin layer of the cream cheese mixture over it. Starting with the short end, roll the salmon up tightly. Repeat this process with the remaining smoked salmon and cream cheese filling. Trim the edges and cut each roll into ½-inch-thick slices. The pinwheels can be served immediately or refrigerated, covered, for several hours or overnight. Garnish each pinwheel with a small sprig of fresh dill or parsley, if desired.

EACH SERVING PROVIDES:

1g carbohydrates, 100 calories, 7g protein, 8g fat,
0g dietary fiber, 313mg sodium, 27mg cholesterol

Smoked Trout Mousse on Cucumber Rounds

These luscious bites of savory smoked trout mousse paired with cucumbers can be served simply by putting a dollop of trout mousse on each cucumber round. To dress up these tasty morsels, place the mousse in a cake decorating bag fitted with a star tip, pipe onto the cucumber rounds, and garnish with a small sprig of parsley or dill. The trout mousse also can be decoratively piped onto the base of trimmed and separated Belgian endive leaves.

4 SERVINGS

2 green onions, cut into 2-inch lengths

$\frac{1}{2}$ pound smoked trout, skin removed and broken into small pieces

4 ounces cream cheese, at room temperature

2 ounces (4 tablespoons) butter, at room temperature

3 tablespoons fresh dill, plus some for garnish

2 tablespoons sour cream

1 tablespoon horseradish

1 tablespoon fresh lemon juice

$\frac{1}{8}$ teaspoon coarse salt

$\frac{1}{8}$ teaspoon freshly ground pepper

1 English (hothouse or seedless) cucumber, cut into $\frac{1}{4}$-inch-thick slices*

PLACE the green onion in the work bowl of a food processor fitted with a metal blade (or in a blender) and process until finely chopped. Add the trout, cream cheese, and butter and blend well. Add the dill, sour cream, horseradish, lemon juice, salt, and pepper and process until smooth.

(continues)

---

*I prefer to use an English cucumber because it is almost seedless. The common variety of cucumber can be substituted, however.

Spoon the smoked trout mousse into a pastry bag (or you can use a freezer bag by cutting one of the corners) fitted with a ½-inch star tip. Pipe generous-size rosettes onto each cucumber round. Garnish with a bit of fresh dill or parsley, if desired. The cucumber rounds can be prepared 4 hours ahead. Place them in a rimmed pan that is higher than the rosettes, cover with plastic wrap, and refrigerate.

EACH SERVING PROVIDES:

4g carbohydrates, 335 calories, 19g protein, 27g fat,
1g dietary fiber, 1285mg sodium, 113mg cholesterol

ABOUT ENGLISH CUCUMBERS

• •

English (hothouse or seedless) cucumbers are long, slender, firm cucumbers with a dark green skin. They are wrapped in plastic shrink-wrap to protect their tender, unwaxed, edible skin, and also to prevent any loss of moisture or crispness. When choosing an English cucumber, look for one that is heavy for its size with a uniformly dark green skin. Store it in the refrigerator in its original wrap and be sure to keep it separate from tomatoes.

Tapenade

Tapenade is a Mediterranean olive spread that has become very popular in recent years. It makes a wonderful spread to serve with low-carbohydrate crackers or vegetables, or, for a savory treat, it can be spread under the skin of chicken before it is baked.

8 SERVINGS

1 clove garlic
1 cup Kalamata olives, pitted and drained
½ cup capers, rinsed and drained

5 anchovies, drained
2 tablespoons extra virgin olive oil
1 teaspoon fresh lemon juice

PLACE the garlic in the work bowl of a food processor fitted with a metal blade (or in a blender) and process until finely chopped. Add the rest of the ingredients and process until the mixture forms a paste. Transfer the tapenade to a covered dish and refrigerate until needed.

EACH SERVING PROVIDES:
3g carbohydrates, 117 calories, 1g protein, 11g fat,
0g dietary fiber, 869mg sodium, 2mg cholesterol

chapter five

STARTLING
SOUPS

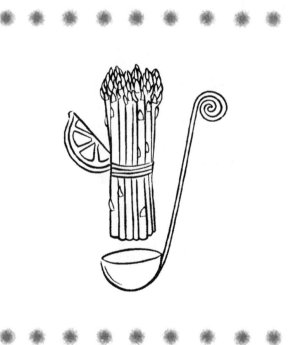

SOUPS

Broccoli Soup

Cabbage and Cheese Soup

Chilled Avocado Soup

Chinese Cucumber and Pork
  Soup

Creamed Spinach Soup

Curried Broccoli Soup

Curried Cauliflower Soup

Curried Crab Soup

Mexican Cheese Soup

Mushroom and Green Onion
  Soup

Savory Spinach Soup

Savory Zucchini Soup

Senegalese Soup

Spicy Roasted Red Pepper
  Soup

Spinach and Bacon Soup

Springtime Asparagus Soup

Tarragon-Infused Celery Soup

Zesty Zucchini Soup

SOUPS ARE ONE OF the most "startling" versatile meals. There are an infinite number of combinations and ways to serve soup, limited only by your imagination. On hot, sultry days during the lazy days of summer, I can think of nothing more refreshing than a mug brimming with chilled soup. At the other extreme, when the temperature outside befits Siberia more than Hawaii, imagine how warming a steamy bowl of hot, flavorful soup can be.

Soups are especially appealing because they are satisfying, hearty, and mouth-watering all at the same time. Some of the best-tasting soups, like Zesty Zucchini Soup, are made with seasonal produce, but most are equally possible year-round. If you are looking for a heartier bowl of soup, then Curried Crab Soup is destined to become one of your favorites. Do you prefer chilled soup no matter what the temperature is outside? Try Chilled Avocado Soup—it's my favorite.

In fact, as you try the various soup recipes, you will soon discover that many of them can be served hot, at room temperature, or chilled—it is strictly a taste preference. Now you see why I say that soups are so versatile. They can be served at any temperature, made early in the day or a day ahead, thinned by adding more liquid, or thickened by adding more ingredients. Almost any soup can be made-to-order.

A word of caution: There are many highly desirable soup ingredients, such as potatoes, corn, and squash, that we traditionally identify as classical components of soup. These vegetables are high in carbohydrates, however, so they must be eliminated from the list of soup ingredients. Also, flour, one of the primary ingredients used to thicken soup, is definitely not on our list of acceptable food items for a low-carbohydrate diet. You can still make a perfectly delectable soup, though, by carefully selecting only those foods allowed on your individual diet plan, combining them with the right herbs and seasoning, and enhancing the thickness with additional low-carbohydrate ingredients, leftover pureed vegetables, or even a beaten egg or two. Just finish off the soup with a garnish of chopped fresh chives, grated cheese, or a few croutons (if permitted), and you can enjoy a soup for every season and at any time of the day. Soup's on!

Broccoli Soup

You will be delighted to discover how easy it is to prepare this rich and satisfying soup. It is delicious all year round because it can be savored as a warming soup on cold, blustery days or enjoyed as a chilled soup when the temperature outside is rising.

4 SERVINGS

2 cups fresh broccoli florets
1½ cups chicken broth
½ cup chopped yellow onion
½ teaspoon dried thyme leaves
½ teaspoon coarse salt
¼ teaspoon freshly ground
   pepper

⅛ teaspoon garlic powder
1 cup buttermilk
4 steamed broccoli florets
   tied with a pimiento strip
   (optional)

COMBINE the broccoli, chicken broth, onion, thyme, salt, pepper, and garlic powder in a large saucepan over medium-high heat and bring to a boil. Cover, and simmer over low heat for 10 minutes. Remove the saucepan from the heat and allow the soup to cool for 10 minutes.

Using a slotted spoon, transfer the broccoli (reserve the liquid in the saucepan) to the work bowl of a food processor fitted with a metal blade (or in a blender) and process until finely chopped. Add the liquid from the saucepan and puree. Add the buttermilk and blend well. (If you do not have a large work bowl, you may have to process the soup in two batches.) Return the soup to the saucepan to reheat. Taste for seasoning.

(continues)

To serve, ladle the soup into four soup bowls and garnish each serving with a steamed broccoli floret tied with a red pimiento strip, if desired.

EACH SERVING PROVIDES:

8g carbohydrates, 52 calories, 4g protein, 1g fat,
2g dietary fiber, 696mg sodium, 4mg cholesterol

ABOUT BROCCOLI

Broccoli is an excellent source of calcium as well as being exceptionally high in the important antioxidants vitamins C and E and a host of other cancer-fighting phytochemicals. This versatile vegetable is a member of the cruciferous family and can be eaten raw, cooked, or even juiced.

When choosing broccoli, look for bunches that have tightly closed green clusters, firm stalks, and a fresh broccoli aroma rather than a cabbage smell. Avoid any with yellow florets, ends that are dried, or woody stems. Wash the broccoli well and, when dry, store in an airtight plastic bag in the refrigerator.

Cabbage and Cheese Soup

Cabbage is not one of my family's favorite vegetables, but whenever I make this soup, they always seem to ask for more.

4 SERVINGS

4 slices bacon, coarsely chopped
½ cup coarsely chopped yellow
  onion
½ cup thinly sliced celery
8 ounces cabbage, thinly sliced
3 cups chicken broth
½ teaspoon coarse salt
½ teaspoon freshly ground
  pepper
¼ teaspoon (or more) cayenne
  pepper
½ cup (or more) grated
  Gruyere or Swiss cheese

LIGHTLY coat a large saucepan with a nonstick vegetable spray and place it over medium heat. Add the bacon and sauté until crisp, stirring occasionally. Add the onion and celery and continue to cook for 4 minutes, stirring occasionally. Add the cabbage, chicken broth, salt, pepper, and cayenne and bring to a boil over medium-high heat. Cover, and simmer over low heat for 15 minutes. Gradually add the cheese and stir until it melts. Taste for seasoning. Ladle the soup into four soup bowls and serve.

EACH SERVING PROVIDES:
7g carbohydrates, 199 calories, 12g protein, 14g fat,
2g dietary fiber, 1377mg sodium, 31mg cholesterol

ABOUT CABBAGE

Cabbage is considered the most ancient of cultivated leafy plants. A member of the cruciferous family, it is related to Brussels sprouts, broccoli, kale, and cauliflower, to name a few. There are three kinds of cabbage, each having leaves that grow close together to form a round head. The leaves of the Savoy are wrinkled while those of the white are pale and smooth with raised veins, and the red has leaves similar to the white except they are purplish-red. Cabbage is an excellent source of vitamin C.

When choosing a head of cabbage, look for one with a firm head, heavy for its size, and with closely trimmed stems. Avoid any cabbage that has discoloration of the leaves. Wash the cabbage well and store in the refrigerator.

Chilled Avocado Soup

Avocados also are known as alligator pears. We most often identify them with a zesty guacamole dip, but they also can be used to make extraordinary chilled (or warm) soup. These divine fruits, packed with important nutrients, add a velvety texture and a distinctive yet mild flavor to this heavenly offering.

4 SERVINGS

2 tablespoons canola oil
¼ cup chopped yellow onion
1 clove garlic, minced
2 cups chicken broth
1 cup milk
2 ripe avocados (about 8 ounces each), peeled, pitted, and cubed

1 teaspoon fresh lime juice
½ teaspoon coarse salt
½ teaspoon freshly ground pepper
¼ teaspoon Tabasco sauce or other hot pepper sauce
2 tablespoons chopped fresh chives (optional)

HEAT a large saucepan over medium heat for 2 minutes. Add the oil and swirl the pan to coat the bottom evenly. Add the onion and garlic and sauté for 2 minutes. Add the chicken broth and milk and bring to a boil over medium-high heat. Cover, reduce the heat to low, and simmer for 10 minutes. Remove the saucepan from the heat and set aside for 10 minutes to cool.

Place the avocados, lime juice, salt, pepper, and Tabasco sauce in the large work bowl of a food processor fitted with a metal blade (or in a blender) and process until finely chopped. Gradually add the chicken broth mixture and blend until smooth. Transfer the soup to a large bowl. Cover, and refrigerate for several hours or overnight. (If serving the soup warm, serve immediately.) To serve, ladle the soup into four soup bowls and garnish with chives, if desired.

(continues)

EACH SERVING PROVIDES:

12g carbohydrates, 271 calories, 5g protein, 24g fat,
5g dietary fiber, 791mg sodium, 8mg cholesterol

HOW TO RIPEN AN AVOCADO

The easiest and quickest way to ripen an avocado is simply to place it in a wool sock and keep it in a dark, enclosed closet or pantry for two days. Once ripened, the avocado can be stored in the refrigerator vegetable bin for up to two weeks.

Chinese Cucumber and Pork Soup

Although you may doubt that this soup could possibly be easy to prepare, don't let the number of ingredients listed influence your decision. Once the pork marinates for several minutes in one bowl, it is then quickly sautéed in a saucepan. The remaining soup ingredients are gradually added to this same saucepan. After one taste of this sensational soup, you will be glad you were not daunted.

6 SERVINGS

2 tablespoons soy sauce

2 teaspoons rice wine

½ teaspoon Splenda or other artificial sweetener

½ pound lean pork, thinly sliced

2 tablespoons canola oil

6 cups chicken broth

2 green onions, thinly sliced

1 small cucumber, peeled and diced

2 teaspoons Asian sesame oil

½ teaspoon coarse salt

¼ teaspoon freshly ground pepper

1 egg, lightly beaten

COMBINE the soy sauce, rice wine, and Splenda in a small bowl. Add the pork and blend well. Set aside for 15 minutes.

Heat a large saucepan over medium heat for 2 minutes. Add the oil and swirl the pan to coat the bottom evenly. Add the pork and stir-fry for 5 minutes. Add the chicken broth and bring to a boil over medium-high heat. Reduce the heat to medium-low and simmer for 10 minutes. Add the green onions, cucumber, sesame oil, salt, and pepper and blend well. Simmer for an additional 5 minutes. Remove the saucepan from the heat and add the egg, stirring constantly. Taste for seasoning. Ladle the soup into six soup bowls and serve.

EACH SERVING PROVIDES:

3g carbohydrates, 144 calories, 11g protein, 9g fat,

0g dietary fiber, 1554mg sodium, 58mg cholesterol

Creamed Spinach Soup

After one taste of this delicious low-carb spinach soup, you will appreciate Popeye's love for this green vegetable. If you are trying to watch your fat intake, omit the cream and simply add an additional ¼ to ½ cup of chicken broth so you will have enough soup to make four servings.

4 SERVINGS

2 tablespoons butter
¼ cup chopped yellow onion
1¼ pounds prewashed spinach
3 cups chicken broth
¼ teaspoon coarse salt

⅛ teaspoon freshly ground
  pepper
⅛ teaspoon ground nutmeg
¼ cup whipping cream
  (optional)

MELT the butter in a large saucepan over medium-low heat. Add the onion and sauté for 4 minutes, stirring occasionally. Add the spinach, chicken broth, salt, pepper, and nutmeg. Cover, and cook for 30 minutes. Remove the saucepan from the heat and allow the soup to cool for 10 minutes.

Transfer the soup to the large work bowl of a food processor fitted with a metal blade (or in a blender) and process until pureed. (If you do not have a large work bowl, you may have to process the soup in two batches.) Return the soup to the saucepan to reheat. Taste for seasoning.

To serve, ladle the soup into four soup bowls and drizzle cream on top, if desired.

EACH SERVING PROVIDES:
7g carbohydrates, 94 calories, 5g protein, 6g fat,
4g dietary fiber, 997mg sodium, 16mg cholesterol

Curried Broccoli Soup

This spicy soup will make all card-carrying broccoli haters disavow their membership. This delectable soup can be served warm or chilled and even garnished with a dollop of sour cream for added flavor and eye appeal.

6 SERVINGS

2 tablespoons extra virgin olive oil

1 cup coarsely chopped yellow onion

2 packages (10 ounces each) frozen chopped broccoli, partially defrosted

5 cups chicken broth

4 teaspoons curry powder

1 teaspoon coarse salt

½ teaspoon freshly ground pepper

¼ teaspoon dried marjoram leaves

6 tablespoons sour cream, for garnish

HEAT a large saucepan over medium heat for 2 minutes. Add the olive oil and swirl the pan to coat the bottom evenly. Add the onion and sauté for 5 minutes, stirring occasionally. Add the broccoli, chicken broth, curry, salt, pepper, and marjoram and bring to a boil over medium-high heat. Cover, and simmer over low heat for 10 minutes. Remove the saucepan from the heat and allow the soup to cool for 10 minutes.

Using a slotted spoon, transfer the broccoli (reserve the liquid in the saucepan) to the large work bowl of a food processor fitted with a metal blade (or in a blender) and process until finely chopped. Gradually add the liquid from the saucepan and puree. (If you do not have a large work bowl, you may have to process the soup in two batches.) Return the soup to the saucepan to reheat. Taste for seasoning.

(continues)

To serve, ladle the soup into six soup bowls and garnish each serving with a dollop of sour cream, if desired. If serving the soup chilled, transfer it to a covered bowl and refrigerate for several hours or overnight. Stir before serving and taste for seasoning.

EACH SERVING PROVIDES:

9g carbohydrates, 92 calories, 4g protein, 5g fat,

4g dietary fiber, 1190mg sodium, 0mg cholesterol

Curried Cauliflower Soup

This soup is devoted to all cauliflower devotees. If you thought you never liked cauliflower, I promise you that after one taste, this soup will soon become a favorite.

4 SERVINGS

1 tablespoon canola oil
½ cup coarsely chopped yellow onion
1 clove garlic, chopped
1 head cauliflower, broken into small florets
3 cups chicken broth

1 teaspoon curry powder
½ teaspoon ground ginger
½ teaspoon coarse salt
¼ teaspoon freshly ground pepper
¼ cup plain yogurt for garnish

HEAT a large saucepan over medium heat for 2 minutes. Add the oil and swirl the pan to coat the bottom evenly. Add the onion and garlic and sauté for 2 minutes, stirring occasionally. Add the cauliflower and sauté for 3 minutes, stirring occasionally. Add the rest of the ingredients and bring to a boil over medium-high heat. Cover, and simmer over low heat for 15 minutes or until the cauliflower is tender. Remove the saucepan from the heat and allow the soup to cool for 15 minutes.

Using a slotted spoon, transfer the cauliflower (reserve the liquid in the saucepan) to the large work bowl of a food processor fitted with a metal blade (or in a blender) and process until pureed. Add the liquid from the saucepan and mix well. (If you do not have a large work bowl, you may have to process the soup in two batches.) Return the soup to the saucepan to reheat. Taste for seasoning.

To serve, ladle the soup into four soup bowls and garnish with a dollop of plain yogurt, if desired.

EACH SERVING PROVIDES:
11g carbohydrates, 86 calories, 4g protein, 4g fat,
4g dietary fiber, 1047mg sodium, 0mg cholesterol

Curried Crab Soup

Although this soup has more carbohydrates than some of the others found in this cookbook, I think you will agree with me that this is one of the most satisfying and tastiest soups you have ever had the good fortune to indulge in.

4 SERVINGS

3 tablespoons butter
2 tomatoes, chopped
½ cup chopped yellow onion
¼ cup chopped celery
¼ cup minced fresh parsley
2 tablespoons minced green
    bell pepper
1 clove garlic, minced
1 bay leaf
½ teaspoon dried basil
¼ teaspoon dried tarragon
    leaves

1 cup chicken broth
1 cup half-and-half
1 cup lump crabmeat, drained
    and broken up
¼ cup dry white wine
¼ teaspoon fresh lemon juice
⅛ teaspoon dried thyme leaves
1 teaspoon curry powder
½ teaspoon freshly ground
    pepper
¼ teaspoon coarse salt

MELT the butter in a large pot over medium heat. Add the tomatoes, onion, celery, parsley, green pepper, garlic, bay leaf, basil, and tarragon. Cover, and cook for 10 minutes. Add the chicken broth, cover, and cook over medium-low heat for 30 minutes. Remove the pot from the heat and discard the bay leaf. Allow the soup to cool for 10 minutes.

Transfer the soup to the large work bowl of a food processor fitted with a metal blade (or in a blender) and process until smooth. (If you do not have a large work bowl, you may have to process the soup in two batches.) Return the soup to the pot. Add the half-and-half, crabmeat, wine, lemon juice, and thyme and blend well. Cook over medium heat until warm. Add the curry, pepper, and salt and blend well. Taste for seasoning. Ladle the soup into four soup bowls and serve.

Mexican Cheese Soup

Although this hot and spicy soup is perfect fare to serve on a cold, wintry day, it can be savored just as well poolside or on the patio. No matter when you serve this soup, it is certain to become a favorite.

4 SERVINGS

2 tablespoons extra virgin
   olive oil
½ cup diced yellow onion
½ cup diced green bell pepper
16 ounces shredded Monterey
   Jack cheese
3 cups chicken broth
1 can (4.5 ounces) chopped
   green chiles

½ teaspoon dried oregano
   leaves
½ teaspoon ground cumin
¼ teaspoon coarse salt
⅛ teaspoon (or more) cayenne
   pepper

HEAT a medium saucepan over medium heat for 2 minutes. Add the olive oil and swirl the pan to coat the bottom evenly. Add the onion and green pepper and sauté for 4 minutes. Add the rest of the ingredients and bring to a boil. Reduce the heat to low and simmer for 10 minutes or just until the cheese melts. Ladle the soup into four soup bowls and serve.

EACH SERVING PROVIDES:

6g carbohydrates, 515 calories, 29g protein, 42g fat,

1g dietary fiber, 1563mg sodium, 101mg cholesterol

Mushroom and Green Onion Soup

Served in mugs, this soup lends itself to casual dining, but it is easily transformed into more elegant fare when presented in a china bowl. No matter how you serve this flavorful offering, you will want to make it part of your prominent culinary repertoire.

4 SERVINGS

8 ounces fresh mushrooms, cleaned and stems trimmed
1 bunch green onions, trimmed
2 tablespoons unsalted butter
¼ teaspoon coarse salt
¼ teaspoon freshly ground pepper
⅛ teaspoon cayenne pepper
3 cups chicken broth
¼ cup sour cream, for garnish

COARSELY chop the mushrooms (thinly slice and reserve two mushrooms). Transfer the chopped mushrooms to a bowl and set aside.

Cut the green onions into 2-inch lengths (thinly slice and reserve one green onion for garnish).

Melt the butter in a large saucepan over medium heat. When it begins to foam, add the chopped green onions, salt, pepper, and cayenne. Cover, and cook over low heat for 10 minutes, stirring occasionally.

Add the chicken broth and whisk over medium-high heat until the soup comes to a boil. Reduce heat to medium-low and simmer, uncovered, for 10 minutes, stirring occasionally. Add the chopped mushrooms and heat thoroughly, about 2 minutes.

Using a slotted spoon, transfer the cooked vegetables (reserve the liquid in the saucepan) to the large work bowl of a food processor fitted with a metal blade (or in a blender) and process for about 1 minute or until pureed. (If you do not have a large work bowl, you may have to process the soup in two batches.)

(continues)

Return the pureed vegetables to the reserved liquid in the saucepan and use a wire whisk to blend well. Add the reserved sliced mushrooms to the soup and cook for 2 minutes.

To serve, ladle the soup into four soup bowls and garnish each serving with a dollop of sour cream and a sprinkling of the reserved sliced green onion.

EACH SERVING PROVIDES:

4g carbohydrates, 76 calories, 2g protein, 6g fat,

1g dietary fiber, 889mg sodium, 16mg cholesterol

Savory Spinach Soup

This is definitely a man's soup, but ladies, you're encouraged to sample it as well. It has a lot more bite than the Creamed Spinach Soup (page 88), yet both are equally tasty.

3 SERVINGS

1 cup water
1 package (1 pound) prewashed spinach
1 tablespoon extra virgin olive oil
2 green onions, coarsely chopped
2 cloves garlic, chopped

2 cups chicken broth
1 teaspoon fresh lemon juice
½ teaspoon dried thyme leaves
½ teaspoon coarse salt
½ teaspoon freshly ground pepper
Pinch ground nutmeg
¼ cup sour cream

BRING 1 cup water to a boil in a pot over high heat. Add the spinach and cook, covered, over low heat for 3 to 4 minutes or until the spinach is wilted. Transfer the spinach to a colander and drain well. When the spinach is cool enough to handle, place it in a towel and squeeze out as much moisture as possible. (The spinach can be prepared a day ahead. Place in a covered container and refrigerate.)

Heat a large saucepan over moderate heat for 2 minutes. Add the olive oil and swirl the pan to coat the bottom evenly. Add the green onions and garlic and sauté for 4 minutes, stirring occasionally. Add the spinach, chicken broth, lemon juice, thyme, salt, pepper, and nutmeg and blend. Bring to a boil over medium-high heat. Cover, and simmer over low heat for 15 minutes. Remove the saucepan from the heat and allow the soup to cool for 10 minutes.

Transfer the soup to the large work bowl of a food processor fitted with a metal blade (or in a blender) and process until pureed. Add the sour cream and blend well. (If you do not have a large work bowl, you

(continues)

may have to process the soup in two batches.) Return the soup to the saucepan to reheat. Taste for seasoning. Ladle the soup into three soup bowls and serve.

Savory Zucchini Soup

When your garden is overflowing with zucchini, you will be delighted to be able to use them in this delectable soup that is bursting with flavors. I prefer to serve the soup plain, but it also can be served with a dollop of yogurt.

3 TO 4 SERVINGS

1 tablespoon butter	$\frac{1}{2}$ teaspoon dried thyme leaves
1 tablespoon extra virgin olive oil	2 cups chicken broth
	$\frac{1}{2}$ teaspoon coarse salt
$\frac{1}{2}$ cup chopped yellow onion	$\frac{1}{4}$ teaspoon freshly ground pepper
$1\frac{1}{4}$ pounds zucchini, thinly sliced	$\frac{1}{4}$ cup plain yogurt (optional)

HEAT the butter and olive oil in a large saucepan over medium heat. When the butter has melted, add the onion and sauté for 4 minutes, stirring occasionally. Add the zucchini and sauté for another 2 minutes, stirring occasionally. Add the thyme and chicken broth. Increase the heat to medium-high and bring to a boil. Cover, and cook over low heat for 30 minutes or until the zucchini is fork-tender. Remove the saucepan from the heat and allow the soup to cool for 10 minutes.

Using a slotted spoon, transfer the zucchini (reserve the liquid in the saucepan) to the large work bowl of a food processor fitted with a metal blade (or in a blender) and process until pureed. (If you do not have a large work bowl, you may have to process the soup in two batches.) Season with salt and pepper and blend well. Return the soup to the saucepan to reheat. Taste for seasoning. Ladle the soup into four soup bowls and top each serving with a dollop of yogurt, if desired.

EACH SERVING PROVIDES:
11g carbohydrates, 145 calories, 5g protein, 10g fat,
3g dietary fiber, 1021mg sodium, 16mg cholesterol

Senegalese Soup

This low-carbohydrate soup can be served hot or chilled. Either way, you will be delighted with the flavor and texture of every spoonful.

6 SERVINGS

4 cups chicken broth
1 cup whipping cream
1 cup sour cream
4 egg yolks
2 teaspoons curry powder
¼ teaspoon celery salt
¼ teaspoon coarse salt
¼ teaspoon fresh lemon juice
⅛ teaspoon cayenne pepper
⅛ teaspoon Worcestershire sauce
1 cup diced cooked chicken breast
Paprika, for garnish
2 to 4 tablespoons chopped fresh chives, for garnish

PLACE the chicken broth in the top of a double boiler and heat over simmering water until it comes almost to a boil. Combine the whipping cream, sour cream, egg yolks, curry, celery salt, salt, lemon juice, cayenne, and Worcestershire sauce in a medium bowl. Using a wire whisk, add ½ cup of the hot chicken broth and blend well. Add this mixture to the chicken broth in the double boiler and cook over simmering water for 15 minutes, stirring constantly until slightly thickened. Remove the double boiler from the heat and cool completely. Refrigerate the soup, covered, for several hours or overnight.

If the soup is to be served warm, reheat it over medium heat. Add the chicken and cook until heated through. Or, if serving the soup chilled, add the chicken to the cold soup. Taste for seasoning.

To serve, ladle the soup into six soup bowls. Sprinkle paprika on each and garnish with chives.

EACH SERVING PROVIDES:

4g carbohydrates, 333 calories, 15g protein, 28g fat,
0g dietary fiber, 904mg sodium, 257mg cholesterol

Spicy Roasted Red Pepper Soup

Roasted peppers add a distinctive taste to this spicy soup. To dress up the soup, spoon the optional saffron cream into a pastry bag fitted with a small tip and pipe a decorative design on top of the soup.

6 SERVINGS

4 red bell peppers
⅓ cup cold water
5 teaspoons minced garlic
5 teaspoons minced fresh
   ginger
1 teaspoon ground cumin
½ teaspoon ground allspice
½ teaspoon ground turmeric
¼ teaspoon dried red pepper
   flakes
2 tablespoons extra virgin
   olive oil
1 cup coarsely chopped yellow
   onions

3 cans (14.5 ounces each)
   fat-free chicken broth
½ teaspoon freshly ground
   pepper
¼ teaspoon coarse salt

Saffron Cream (optional)
⅛ teaspoon saffron threads
2 tablespoons warm water
¾ teaspoon finely minced garlic
¾ teaspoon finely minced fresh
   ginger
½ cup sour cream

To roast the red peppers, place them on a baking sheet lined with aluminum foil. Broil the peppers under a preheated broiler, turning the peppers as the skin blackens, for 20 minutes or until the skins are charred all over. Once the peppers are roasted, place them in a plastic bag, seal, and allow them to steam for 15 to 20 minutes. When the peppers are cool enough to handle, peel away the skin and remove the top and seeds. (Do not rinse the peppers.)

Put the water, 5 teaspoons garlic, 5 teaspoons ginger, cumin, allspice, turmeric, and red pepper flakes in the work bowl of a food processor fitted with a metal blade (or in a blender) and process until well blended.

(continues)

Heat a large saucepan over medium-low heat for 2 minutes. Add the olive oil and swirl the pan to coat the bottom evenly. Add the onion, cover, and cook for 15 minutes, stirring occasionally. Increase the heat to medium-high and add the spice mixture. Cook, uncovered, for 5 minutes, stirring frequently. Add the chicken broth, pepper, and salt and bring to a boil. Reduce the heat to medium-low and simmer for 25 minutes. Remove the saucepan from the heat and allow the soup to cool for 10 minutes.

While the soup is cooling, make the optional Saffron Cream by dissolving the saffron threads in 2 tablespoons warm water. Coat a small nonstick skillet with a nonstick vegetable spray and place over medium heat for 1 minute. Add the ¾ teaspoon garlic and ¾ teaspoon ginger and sauté for 1 minute, stirring frequently. Add the saffron mixture and cook for 1 minute. Remove the saucepan from the heat, add the sour cream, and blend well. Set aside. (The Saffron Cream can be made a day ahead. Cover the saucepan and refrigerate. Bring to room temperature before serving.)

Place the red peppers in the work bowl of a food processor fitted with a metal blade (or in a blender) and process until pureed. Add the soup mixture and process until smooth. (If you do not have a large work bowl, you may have to process the soup in two batches.) Return the soup to the saucepan to reheat. Taste for seasoning.

To serve, ladle the soup into six soup bowls. Spoon the Saffron Cream into a pastry bag (or you can use a freezer bag by cutting one of the corners) fitted with a small writing tip and pipe a cobweb, concentric circles, or random lines across each serving of soup, if desired.

EACH SERVING PROVIDES:
11g carbohydrates, 95 calories, 2g protein, 5g fat,
2g dietary fiber, 971mg sodium, 0mg cholesterol

Spinach and Bacon Soup

One of the best things about being on a low-carbohydrate diet is that you don't have to feel guilty when enjoying bacon. It lends a wonderful flavor to this hearty soup and is a nice complement to the spinach as well.

6 SERVINGS

4 slices bacon, diced, plus 2
   slices, crumbled for garnish
½ cup coarsely chopped yellow
   onion
½ cup coarsely chopped celery
6 cups prewashed spinach
6 cups chicken broth

1 teaspoon freshly ground
   pepper
½ teaspoon coarse salt
¾ cup whipping cream
2 egg yolks
2 slices crumbled cooked
   bacon, for garnish

LIGHTLY coat a large saucepan with a nonstick vegetable spray and place over medium heat for 1 minute. Add the bacon and sauté for 2 minutes, stirring occasionally. Reduce the heat to medium low and add the onion and celery. Sauté for 4 minutes, stirring occasionally. Add the spinach, broth, pepper, and salt and bring to a boil over medium-high heat. Cover, and simmer over low heat for 15 minutes. Remove the saucepan from the heat and allow the soup to cool for 10 minutes.

Transfer the soup to the large work bowl of a food processor fitted with a metal blade (or in a blender) and process until pureed. (If you do not have a large work bowl, you may have to process the soup in two batches.) Return the soup to the saucepan.

Combine the whipping cream and egg yolks in a small bowl and blend well. Slowly add this mixture to the soup and stir well. Cook over medium heat for 7 to 10 minutes or just until the soup is heated

(continues)

through, stirring frequently. (Do not let the soup come to a boil or the egg yolks will curdle.) Taste for seasoning.

To serve, ladle the soup into six soup bowls and garnish each serving with crumbled bacon, if desired.

EACH SERVING PROVIDES:
5g carbohydrates, 171 calories, 5g protein, 15g fat,
1g dietary fiber, 1301mg sodium, 115mg cholesterol

Springtime Asparagus Soup

Although asparagus is available year-round now, I still have fond memories of seeing asparagus bundles in the supermarket at the first sign of spring. A steaming bowlful of this creamy delight will help you welcome the season.

6 SERVINGS

4 cups chicken broth
2 pounds asparagus spears, cut into 2-inch lengths
1 teaspoon freshly ground pepper
½ teaspoon coarse salt
2 tablespoons extra virgin olive oil

1 large leek, washed and thinly sliced
6 tablespoons sour cream (optional)
6 tablespoons whipping cream, whipped (optional)

BRING the chicken broth to a boil in a medium saucepan over medium heat. Add the asparagus. Cover, and simmer over medium-low heat for 15 minutes. Remove the saucepan from the heat. Add the pepper and salt and blend well. Allow the soup to cool for 10 minutes.

While the asparagus is cooling, heat a small skillet over medium heat for 1 minute. Add the olive oil and swirl it in the pan to coat the bottom evenly. Add the leek and sauté for 3 to 4 minutes or until tender.

Using a slotted spoon, transfer the asparagus (reserve the liquid in the saucepan) to the large work bowl of a food processor fitted with a metal blade (or in a blender). Add the leek and process until pureed. Add the reserved liquid and process until smooth. (If you do not have a large work bowl, you may have to process the soup in two batches.) Return the soup to the saucepan to reheat. Taste for seasoning.

(continues)

To serve, ladle the soup into six soup bowls. Garnish with a dollop of sour cream or whipping cream, if desired.

EACH SERVING PROVIDES:
9g carbohydrates, 91 calories, 4g protein, 5g fat,
3g dietary fiber, 844mg sodium, 0mg cholesterol

Tarragon-Infused Celery Soup

When just a tiny amount of tarragon is added to this soup, it heightens the flavor of celery. I like to serve the soup piping hot, but it's equally delicious when served chilled. Simply add ¼ cup milk and ¼ cup whipping cream after the soup is pureed, and then refrigerate it for several hours or overnight.

4 SERVINGS

1 tablespoon extra virgin olive oil	2 cups chicken broth
2 cups thinly sliced celery	½ teaspoon coarse salt
½ cup thinly sliced yellow onion	¼ teaspoon freshly ground pepper
2 tablespoons minced fresh parsley	⅛ teaspoon dried tarragon leaves

HEAT a large saucepan over medium heat for 2 minutes. Add the olive oil and swirl the pan to coat the bottom evenly. Add the celery, onion, and parsley and sauté for 5 minutes, stirring occasionally. Add the rest of the ingredients and bring to a boil over medium-high heat. Cover, and simmer over low heat for 20 minutes. Remove the saucepan from the heat and allow the soup to cool for 10 minutes.

Using a slotted spoon, transfer the vegetable mixture (reserve the liquid in the saucepan) to the large work bowl of a food processor fitted with a metal blade (or in a blender) and process until pureed. Add the liquid from the saucepan and mix until well blended. (If you do not have a large work bowl, you may have to process the soup in two batches.) Return the soup to the saucepan to reheat. Taste for seasoning. Ladle the soup into four soup bowls and serve.

EACH SERVING PROVIDES:

4g carbohydrates, 53 calories, 1g protein, 4g fat, 1g dietary fiber, 800mg sodium, 0mg cholesterol

Zesty Zucchini Soup

I like to cook zucchini in a fragrant chicken broth for added flavor. Once the zucchini is cooked and pureed, all of the chicken broth can be added. However, I prefer soups that are thick, so I add just enough broth to the zucchini to create a richly satisfying and dense soup. If all the broth is added, the soup will serve four people.

3 SERVINGS

1 pound zucchini, cut into cubes
3 cups chicken broth
½ teaspoon curry powder
½ teaspoon ground ginger
½ teaspoon ground cinnamon
¼ teaspoon coarse salt
¼ teaspoon freshly ground pepper
½ cup sour cream
2 to 3 tablespoons toasted almonds, for garnish*

COMBINE the zucchini, chicken broth, curry, ginger, cinnamon, salt, and pepper in a large saucepan over medium-high heat and bring to a boil. Cover, and simmer over low heat for 15 minutes. Remove the saucepan from the heat and allow the soup to cool for 10 minutes.

Using a slotted spoon, transfer the zucchini (reserve the liquid in the saucepan) to the large work bowl of a food processor fitted with a metal blade (or in a blender) and process until pureed. Add just enough reserved liquid to the zucchini until the soup is the desired consistency. Add the sour cream and lightly blend. (If you do not have a large work bowl, you may have to process the soup in two batches.) Return the soup to the saucepan to reheat. Taste for seasoning.

To serve, ladle the soup into three soup bowls and garnish with almond slivers, if desired.

EACH SERVING PROVIDES:
8g carbohydrates, 115 calories, 4g protein, 7g fat,
2g dietary fiber, 1204mg sodium, 33mg cholesterol

*To toast the almonds: Preheat oven to 350 degrees F. Place the almonds in a shallow pan and bake for 10 to 15 minutes or until golden brown.

chapter six

SAVVY
SALADS

* * * * * * * *

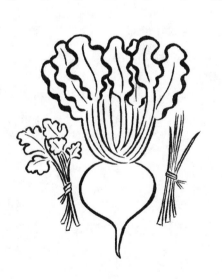

* * * * * * * *

SALADS

Main Event Salads

Beef Fajita Salad

Chef's Salad

Classic Chicken Salad

Cobb Chicken Salad

Curried Chicken Salad

Fresh Flounder Salad

Italian Beef Salad

Marinated Tofu and Mixed
    Baby Greens

Poached Salmon Salad

Pork Tenderloin and Goat
    Cheese Salad

Savory Spinach Salad with
    Steak and Blue Cheese

Shrimp and Feta Salad

Shrimp and Mushroom Salad

Tarragon Chicken Salad

Green with Envy Salads

Asparagus and Walnut Salad

Caesar Salad

Cauliflower (sans Potato) Salad

Greek Salad

Mixed Baby Greens with Blue
    Cheese and Walnuts

Mixed Baby Greens, Endive,
    Roquefort, and Walnut
    Salad

Mixed Baby Greens with Goat
    Cheese

Mixed Baby Greens with
    Shallot Vinaigrette

Mixed Baby Greens with
    Tarragon-Scented
    Vinaigrette

Old-Fashioned Coleslaw

Romaine Salad with Romano
    Cheese

Spinach Salad with Bacon

Spinach Salad with Blue
    Cheese Vinaigrette

Spinach Salad with Maytag
    Blue Cheese

THE SALAD HAS BEEN an essential component of a good meal for centuries. Ancient Romans enjoyed *herba salata,* or "salted greens." While the Colosseum crowd dressed their simple greens with only oil, vinegar, and a few herbs, in the new millennium, salads have evolved into an artful cornucopia of tastes, colors, and textures, brimming with an interesting assortment of greens and adorned with a variety of traditional and exotic vegetables. In many kitchens today, salads have been elevated to main course salad status by simply adding beef, poultry, seafood, or cheese to the greens.

When we think of a salad, the first ingredients that come to mind are the greens. These leafy vegetables are the foundation of most salads, and although they are most often green in color, some are red or white instead. For this reason, greens not only add flavor and texture to salads, they also can contribute an interesting variety of colors.

When shopping for salad greens, make sure they are as fresh as possible. Look for greens with fresh, crisp leaves, a garden-fresh aroma, and a just-plucked appearance. Avoid any greens that are spotted with brown marks or have oversized wilted leaves.

Many of the popular varieties can be found prewashed in cellophane bags. If you cannot find the greens of your choice or prefer to buy loose lettuce, you will have to wash and dry the greens before using them in a salad. The method I like is simply to tear each leaf along the middle of the central rib, or tear into generous bite-size pieces. The large pieces maintain crispness so the greens don't lose their crunch, and they also look more attractive in a salad.

After the leaves are prepared, immerse them either in a sink or a pot filled with cold water and swish them around with your hands or rinse under cold running water to remove any grit.

Once the leaves are washed, the next step is to dry them. This step is very important because if the leaves are not completely dry, the vinaigrettes used to dress them can become diluted and the salad will not taste as good as it should. This is also a good time to discard any leaves that are brown or wilted. As you lift the leaves from the water, gently shake them to remove as much water as possible. One way of drying the greens is to place them in a pillowcase, tightly secured at the neck, and swing the bag in a circle outdoors. My favorite way is to put the pillowcase in the washing machine and turn on the "spin" cycle; I often run this cycle twice. Of course, a kitchen salad spinner is one of the best ways to dry lettuce.

When the greens are washed and dried, they are ready to be made into a delectable salad. If you are not going to use them right away, simply place the leaves in a salad crisper or wrap them loosely in a cloth or paper towel. Roll up the towel and place it in a plastic bag. Poke holes in the plastic bag to allow any excess moisture to escape. Greens can be stored in the refrigerator this way for 4 or 5 days.

Now that the greens are properly prepared, you are almost ready to venture into the world of savvy salads. But before you do, keep in mind that the crowning touch to any good salad is the vinaigrette. The more robust or assertive a vinaigrette, the more certain you can be that the salad you prepare will be highly flavorful and pleasing to the palate. Although I provide recipes for a wide variety of vinaigrettes, an impressive array of excellent commercial vinaigrettes and salad dressings is available in most supermarkets and gourmet shops. So, whether you are hungry for a robust salad, such as Spinach Salad with Bacon, or in the mood for a more elegant one, such as Mixed Baby Greens, Endive, Roquefort, and Walnut Salad, you are certain to be pleased. After you have had a chance to sample some of the salad creations found in this chapter, I hope you will agree that salads have grown up.

* * * * * * * * *

MAIN EVENT SALADS

A salad is not only appropriate as one of several courses comprising a meal—it can be the entire meal. Complementing a variety of greens with a well-chosen portion of poultry, meat, or seafood can elevate this garden bounty to main course status.

Beef Fajita Salad

This savory main course salad consists of a marinated flank steak and vinaigrette that are richly imbued with the distinctive flavors of the Southwest and complemented with traditional fajita fixings. Even without the tortilla, this salad is the closest thing to eating a beef fajita.

4 SERVINGS

½ cup extra virgin olive oil

2 tablespoons white wine vinegar

1 clove garlic, minced

1⅛ teaspoons ground cumin

1 teaspoon chili powder

½ teaspoon coarse salt

½ teaspoon freshly ground pepper

¼ teaspoon cayenne pepper

1 large red bell pepper *use raw*

6 cups romaine lettuce, broken into generous bite-size pieces

1½ pounds Tex-Mex Flank Steak (page 214) or favorite cooked beef, thinly sliced

4 ounces Monterey Jack cheese, cut into cubes *or shredded*

1 avocado, peeled and cubed

~~¼ cup sour cream~~ *red onion slices*

To make the Southwestern Vinaigrette, combine the olive oil, vinegar, garlic, cumin, chili powder, salt, pepper, and cayenne in a small jar with a tight-fitting lid.* Shake well to blend. Set aside.

To roast the red pepper, place it on a baking sheet lined with aluminum foil. Broil it under a preheated broiler, turning the pepper as the skin blackens, for 20 minutes or until the skin is charred all over. Once the pepper is roasted, place it in a plastic bag, seal, and allow it to steam for 15 to 20 minutes. When the pepper is cool enough to handle, peel away the skin and remove the top and seeds. (Do not rinse the pepper.) Cut the pepper into thin slices.

*Commercial southwestern dressings or vinaigrettes can be substituted for the Southwestern Vinaigrette.

To serve, make a bed of the romaine lettuce on each of four dinner plates. Arrange overlapping slices of flank steak on the lettuce and randomly distribute the pepper, cheese, and avocado over the top. Spoon a dollop of sour cream in the center of each salad and drizzle Southwestern Vinaigrette over all.

EACH SERVING PROVIDES:

10g carbohydrates, 850 calories, 57g protein, 64g fat,
5g dietary fiber, 557mg sodium, 152mg cholesterol

Chef's Salad

A chef's salad is one of the most versatile all-time favorites. It can be made with a variety of meats, cheeses, and greens and dressed with Thousand Island dressing, Italian Vinaigrette (page 123), or whatever you fancy.

4 SERVINGS

3 cups romaine lettuce, torn into generous bite-size pieces

3 ounces prewashed spinach, trimmed

6 ounces cooked turkey breast or chicken breast, cut into ¼-inch strips

4 ounces baked ham, cut into ¼-inch strips

4 ounces Swiss cheese, cut into ¼-inch strips

2 hard-boiled eggs, peeled and quartered

Favorite dressing or vinaigrette

COMBINE the lettuce, spinach, turkey, ham, cheese, and eggs in a large salad bowl. Add just enough dressing to bind the ingredients together; lightly blend.

To serve, arrange the salad on each of four dinner plates, dividing evenly among the servings.

EACH SERVING PROVIDES:

3g carbohydrates, 293 calories, 32g protein, 16g fat, 1g dietary fiber, 164mg sodium, 176mg cholesterol

Classic Chicken Salad

Whether you are serving this salad for lunch or dinner, you will be delighted with its complexity of flavors, texture, and ingredients.

4 SERVINGS

4 cups cubed cooked chicken breasts (or crabmeat)*

2 celery ribs, thinly sliced

½ cup thinly sliced green onion

⅓ cup chopped fresh parsley

½ teaspoon coarse salt

¼ teaspoon freshly ground pepper

¼ cup fresh lemon juice

¼ cup extra virgin olive oil

1 cup (or more) mayonnaise

½ to 1 cup chopped walnuts (optional)

COMBINE the chicken, celery, green onion, parsley, salt, and pepper in a medium bowl and lightly blend.

Combine the lemon juice and olive oil in a small bowl and blend well. Pour this mixture over the chicken salad and mix well. Let the chicken salad sit for at least 30 minutes to allow the flavors to steep.

Add just enough mayonnaise to bind the ingredients together; lightly blend. Add the optional walnuts. Taste for seasoning.

To serve, spoon the salad on each of four dinner plates, dividing evenly among the servings.

EACH SERVING PROVIDES:

5g carbohydrates, 900 calories, 45g protein, 77g fat, 2g dietary fiber, 678mg sodium, 165mg cholesterol

*To cook chicken breasts: Preheat oven to 350 degrees F. Place the chicken breasts in a shallow pan and cover with a piece of aluminum foil. Bake for 25 to 30 minutes. Or, the chicken breasts can be placed in a large saucepan filled with boiling water and poached for 10 minutes. Turn off the heat and leave the saucepan on the burner. Allow the chicken breasts to come to room temperature. Drain well. Pat dry.

Cobb Chicken Salad

Cobb salad was made famous by Bob Cobb's Brown Derby restaurant in Los Angeles, California. It is traditionally made with tomatoes, but I have omitted them to keep the carbohydrate content to a minimum.

4 SERVINGS

½ cup extra virgin olive oil

¼ cup balsamic vinegar

2 teaspoons Dijon mustard

½ teaspoon coarse salt

½ teaspoon freshly ground pepper

6 cups romaine lettuce, torn into bite-size pieces

4 cooked chicken breast halves, thinly sliced

8 slices cooked crispy bacon, crumbled

4 hard-boiled eggs, quartered

6 ounces Maytag Blue Cheese or favorite blue cheese, crumbled

1 avocado, peeled and diced (optional)

To prepare the Balsamic Vinaigrette, combine the olive oil, vinegar, mustard, salt, and pepper in a jar with a tight-fitting lid.* Shake until well blended. Refrigerate until needed. Shake well before using and taste for seasoning.

To prepare the Cobb salad, place the lettuce, chicken, bacon, eggs, cheese, and optional avocado in a large salad bowl and lightly toss. Add enough Balsamic Vinaigrette to make the lettuce leaves glisten, and toss again.

*Commercial blue cheese dressing or any of your favorite salad dressings can be substituted for the Balsamic Vinaigrette.

To serve, arrange the salad on each of four dinner plates, dividing evenly among the servings.

EACH SERVING PROVIDES:

10g carbohydrates, 777 calories, 48g protein, 60g fat,
4g dietary fiber, 1242mg sodium, 298mg cholesterol

ABOUT BALSAMIC VINEGAR

Balsamic vinegar is a highly aromatic vinegar that is produced in and around the Modena region of Italy. It is made by gently crushing the white Trebbiano grape, or other choice grapes, to release the tannins in their skin, and then simmering the juice until about 25 percent of the liquid evaporates. This sweet grape syrup is then poured into fragrant wooden casks and left for a year.

During this time, air space is left in the wooden casks for oxidation, and slowly, wine yeast feeds on the sugar and converts it to alcohol. At the same time, but much more slowly, acetic bacteria consumes the alcohol and transforms it into acetic acid.

Because the sugar is too high for the yeast to consume, what remains sweetens the vinegar.

As the volume decreases through evaporation, the vinegar is transferred to a succession of increasingly smaller, fragrant wooden casks for 6 to 120 years, and sometimes even longer. The longer balsamic vinegar ages, the more mellow, and the more expensive, it becomes.

Although balsamic vinegar is traditionally red in color, it is now available in a pale, clear color with a lighter taste.

Curried Chicken Salad

This salad is so delightfully tasty you may want to double the ingredients so you can enjoy it the following day. In fact, the salad tastes best if made one day before serving to allow the flavors to blend.

6 SERVINGS

1 clove garlic
¼ teaspoon chopped fresh ginger
3 tablespoons fresh lemon juice
1 teaspoon curry powder
1 teaspoon Dijon mustard
¼ teaspoon coarse salt
¼ teaspoon freshly ground pepper
½ cup canola oil

3 to 4 cups cooked and cubed chicken
2 cups broccoli florets, blanched (or plunged into boiling water) for 1 minute
1¼ cups sliced celery
¾ cup salted cashews (optional)
6 cups prewashed spinach
Chives, for garnish

To make the Curry Vinaigrette, place the garlic and ginger in the work bowl of a food processor fitted with a metal blade (or in a blender) and process until finely chopped. Add the lemon juice, curry, mustard, salt, and pepper and blend. Pour the canola oil in a slow, steady stream and process until smooth. (The vinaigrette can be made a day ahead. Transfer it to a covered container and refrigerate until 1 hour before serving. When ready to use, whisk the vinaigrette and taste for seasoning.)

Combine the chicken, broccoli, celery, and optional cashews in a large bowl. Add the Curry Vinaigrette and toss until well blended.

To serve, make a bed of the spinach on each of six dinner plates. Spoon the salad in the center of the spinach, dividing evenly among the servings. Garnish each serving with long strands of chives randomly placed on the salad, if desired.

EACH SERVING PROVIDES:

5g carbohydrates, 318 calories, 22g protein, 24g fat,
2g dietary fiber, 213mg sodium, 62mg cholesterol

Fresh Flounder Salad

I find this salad to be a refreshing change from the old favorite, tuna salad. This salad also can be made with cod, orange roughy, salmon, or halibut. Whichever fish you use, I think you will agree with me that this is one of the most satisfying salads you have ever tasted.

4 SERVINGS

1½ tablespoons extra virgin
   olive oil
1 pound flounder
¾ cup thinly sliced celery
3 green onions, thinly sliced
2 to 3 tablespoons chopped
   fresh dill (or 1½ tablespoons
   dried dill weed)

½ cup (or less) mayonnaise
½ teaspoon coarse salt
¼ teaspoon freshly ground
   pepper
4 cups red leaf lettuce
4 sprigs of fresh dill, for garnish
   (optional)

HEAT a large nonstick skillet over medium-high heat for 2 minutes. Add the olive oil and swirl the pan to coat the bottom evenly. Add the flounder and sauté for 3 minutes on each side. Transfer the flounder to a large bowl and allow it to cool for 10 minutes.

Break up the flounder and add the celery, green onions, and dill. Add just enough mayonnaise to bind the ingredients together. Season with salt and pepper and lightly blend. Taste for seasoning.

To serve, make a bed of the lettuce leaves on each of four dinner plates and mound the flounder salad in the center, dividing evenly among the servings. Garnish with a sprig of dill, if desired.

EACH SERVING PROVIDES:
3g carbohydrates, 350 calories, 22g protein, 27g fat,
2g dietary fiber, 503mg sodium, 74mg cholesterol

(continues)

Savvy Salads
••••

ABOUT BUYING FISH

When buying fresh fish, look for whole ones that are firm to the touch; have firm, glossy scales; and have bright, clear eyes. Fillets or steaks should have a moist, glossy sheen and a translucent appearance, and the edges should be clean and even. All fish should have a fresh sea smell rather than a fish odor.

To check for doneness when cooking, insert a fork or knife into the thickest part of the fish and determine if the flesh is flaky and no longer translucent. If you are using a meat thermometer, the fish should have an internal temperature of 140 degrees F.

Italian Beef Salad

Pack your picnic hamper with a red-and-white-checkered tablecloth and include an assortment of olives, cheese, and Marinated Artichokes and Mushrooms (page 64), along with this bellisimo salad.

4 SERVINGS

3 tablespoons garlic red wine vinegar

1 teaspoon Dijon mustard

½ teaspoon dried basil

½ teaspoon dried oregano leaves

¼ teaspoon coarse salt

¼ teaspoon freshly ground pepper

½ cup extra virgin olive oil

8 ounces beef tenderloin (or favorite beef)

6 cups romaine lettuce, torn into large bite-size pieces

¼ pound provolone cheese, cubed

¼ cup thinly sliced red onion

To make the Italian Vinaigrette, combine the vinegar, mustard, basil, oregano, salt, and pepper in a small bowl and blend well. Gradually whisk in the olive oil until well blended.

Place the beef in a resealable plastic bag and add ¼ cup of the vinaigrette. Turn to coat all over. Seal the bag and refrigerate for several hours or overnight.

Refrigerate the remaining vinaigrette in a covered container until needed. Stir before using and taste for seasoning.

Preheat oven to 400 degrees F. Remove the beef from the marinade (discard the marinade) and place it in a shallow pan. Bake for 40 to 45 minutes or until a meat thermometer registers 145 degrees F. Allow the beef to come to room temperature before cutting into thin slices.

(continues)

To serve, combine the lettuce, beef, cheese, and onion in a large bowl and lightly toss. Add the remaining Italian Vinaigrette and toss well. Arrange the salad on each of four dinner plates, dividing evenly among the servings.

EACH SERVING PROVIDES:

4g carbohydrates, 490 calories, 25g protein, 42g fat,
2g dietary fiber, 442mg sodium, 67mg cholesterol

Marinated Tofu and Mixed Baby Greens

Tofu, or bean curd, is a high-protein soybean food. While it is somewhat bland in taste, when marinated in an Asian-inspired marinade, it readily absorbs the flavors. In addition, the marinated tofu reaches still greater dimensions of tastes when intermingled with mixed baby greens and enlivened with Sherry Vinaigrette.

4 SERVINGS

1½ pounds firm tofu

3 tablespoons soy sauce

1 tablespoon Splenda or other artificial sweetener

1½ tablespoons chopped fresh ginger

2 teaspoons canola oil

1½ teaspoons (or less) Sriracha hot chili sauce or other hot pepper sauce

¾ teaspoon Asian sesame oil

6 cups mixed baby greens

½ red bell pepper, cut into julienne strips

1 recipe Sherry Vinaigrette (page 127) or favorite vinaigrette

PLACE the tofu between two flat plates. Place a bowl filled with water (or one to two 2-pound cans) on the upper plate (there should be just enough weight to make the tofu bulge slightly) and refrigerate for 1 hour.

Drain off any accumulated water from the tofu. Slice the tofu in half horizontally. Set aside.

To make the marinade, combine the soy sauce, Splenda, ginger, canola oil, hot pepper sauce, and sesame oil in a dish and blend well. Place the tofu in the marinade and turn to coat both sides. Cover the dish and refrigerate for 1 to 2 hours, turning the tofu at least once.

(continues)

Transfer the tofu to a shallow baking pan (discard the marinade) and place under a preheated broiler, 3 inches from the heat source, and broil for 4 to 6 minutes on each side or until golden brown. Cut into four pieces.

To serve, make a bed of the mixed baby greens on each of four salad plates. Place a piece of tofu on each and randomly distribute red pepper strips over the top. Drizzle Sherry Vinaigrette over each serving.

EACH SERVING PROVIDES:
9g carbohydrates, 415 calories, 13g protein, 38g fat,
2g dietary fiber, 1077mg sodium, 0mg cholesterol

Poached Salmon Salad

For ease in preparation, I like to poach salmon. I suggest removing the skin before cooking to remove any bacteria that may be hidden there. If you have a friendly butcher, he might be willing to do this simple task for you. Although I prefer the combination of the salmon salad combined with a Sherry Vinaigrette, substituting a raspberry vinaigrette would also nicely complement it, as would any of your other favorite commercial varieties.

4 SERVINGS

½ cup extra virgin olive oil

2 tablespoons sherry vinegar

1 teaspoon Dijon mustard

½ teaspoon coarse salt

¼ teaspoon freshly ground pepper

1½ pounds salmon fillet, skin removed

¼ cup cold water

1 cup thinly sliced celery

½ cup thinly sliced green onion

2 tablespoons capers, rinsed and drained

6 cups mixed baby greens

To make the Sherry Vinaigrette, combine the olive oil, vinegar, mustard, salt, and pepper in the work bowl of a food processor fitted with a metal blade and process until well blended. (A blender or a jar with a tight-fitting lid can be used instead of a food processor; shake well.) Set aside.

Place the salmon in a microwave-safe dish and add ¼ cup water. Cover the dish with plastic wrap. Microwave on high for 8 to 10 minutes or until the salmon is no longer red when a knife is inserted into the thickest part (or a meat thermometer registers 140 degrees F). Allow the salmon to cool to room temperature.

(continues)

Transfer the salmon to a plate. Pat dry with paper towels. Cut the salmon into cubes or flake it. Place the salmon in a large bowl and add the celery, green onion, and capers. Add just enough Sherry Vinaigrette to coat the salad ingredients; lightly blend. Taste for seasoning. To serve, make a bed of mixed baby greens on each of four dinner plates. Spoon the salmon salad in the center of the lettuce, dividing evenly among servings.

EACH SERVING PROVIDES:

2g carbohydrates, 398 calories, 34g protein, 27g fat,
1g dietary fiber, 502mg sodium, 88mg cholesterol

Pork Tenderloin and Goat Cheese Salad

Leftover Better Than Hot Pork Tenderloin is absolutely sensational in this salad, but any of your other favorite pork recipes will do. I also like to use the Walnut Vinaigrette as an accent, but if walnut oil is unavailable, Sesame Vinaigrette (page 132) or Sherry Vinaigrette (page 127) are nice alternatives. Or, don't hesitate to use any of your own commercial favorites.

4 SERVINGS

2 tablespoons red wine vinegar
1½ teaspoons Dijon mustard
¼ teaspoon coarse salt
¼ teaspoon freshly ground pepper
½ cup good-quality walnut oil
6 cups mixed baby greens

1¼ pounds cooked Better Than Hot Pork Tenderloin (page 175) or favorite cooked pork recipe, thinly sliced
4 ounces goat cheese (such as Montrachet), cut into 4 pieces

To make the Walnut Vinaigrette, combine the red wine vinegar, mustard, salt, and pepper in a medium bowl. Gradually whisk in the walnut oil and blend well. Taste for seasoning.

To serve, make a bed of the mixed baby greens on each of four dinner plates. Slightly overlap pork slices on top of greens and place a piece of cheese off to the side. Drizzle Walnut Vinaigrette over each serving.

EACH SERVING PROVIDES:
5g carbohydrates, 614 calories, 43g protein, 47g fat,
2g dietary fiber, 658mg sodium, 121mg cholesterol

Savory Spinach Salad with Steak and Blue Cheese

Although I recommend using the Southwestern Rubbed Flank Steak for its wonderful spicy flavor, you can substitute any of your favorite steak recipes or even a spiced roast beef from the deli. One of your own bottled vinaigrettes also can be substituted for the Balsamic Vinaigrette.

4 SERVINGS

6 cups prewashed spinach
1 recipe Southwestern Rubbed
    Flank Steak (page 209) or
    favorite cooked beef, thinly
    sliced
4 ounces Maytag Blue Cheese
    or favorite blue cheese,
    crumbled

1 red bell pepper, cut into
    julienne strips
2 green onions, thinly sliced
1 recipe Balsamic Vinaigrette
    (page 118)

COMBINE the spinach, flank steak, cheese, red pepper, and green onions in a large bowl. Add just enough Balsamic Vinaigrette to make the spinach leaves glisten. Toss well. To serve, arrange the salad on each of four dinner plates, dividing evenly among the servings.

EACH SERVING PROVIDES:
7g carbohydrates, 407 calories, 44g protein, 22g fat,
3g dietary fiber, 789mg sodium, 109mg cholesterol

Shrimp and Feta Salad

I like to dress this salad with Sherry Vinaigrette, but it also lends itself to adornment by a Greek Vinaigrette (page 142) or whatever else you may fancy. You also can use precooked shrimp if time is of the essence.

4 SERVINGS

1 tablespoon canola oil
1 pound large raw shrimp, peeled and deveined
½ teaspoon coarse salt
¼ teaspoon freshly ground pepper

6 cups mixed baby greens
3 ounces feta cheese, crumbled
1 recipe Sherry Vinaigrette (page 127)
8 pitted Kalamata olives

HEAT a large nonstick skillet over medium-high heat for 1 minute. Add the canola oil and swirl the pan to coat the bottom evenly. Place the shrimp in the skillet and season with salt and pepper. Stir-fry for 1 to 2 minutes or until the shrimp are no longer pink. Remove the skillet from the heat.

Combine the mixed baby greens, shrimp, and cheese in a large bowl and lightly toss. Add enough Sherry Vinaigrette to make the leaves glisten.

To serve, arrange the salad on each of four plates. Garnish each serving with two Kalamata olives.

EACH SERVING PROVIDES:
4g carbohydrates, 488 calories, 28g protein, 39g fat,
2g dietary fiber, 1138mg sodium, 240mg cholesterol

Shrimp and Mushroom Salad

My favorite time to make this exceptional salad is when I have leftover Chinese Shrimp Kebabs. To be certain I have enough shrimp, I always double the recipe. The salad also is delicious when you make it with fresh or precooked shrimp.

4 SERVINGS

1 clove garlic
1½ teaspoons sherry vinegar
1½ teaspoons soy sauce
¼ teaspoon Dijon mustard
⅛ teaspoon coarse salt
⅓ cup peanut or canola oil
2 tablespoons Asian sesame oil
1½ pounds Chinese Shrimp
    Kebabs (page 49) or
    precooked large shrimp

12 fresh button mushrooms,
    thinly sliced
2 green onions, thinly sliced
6 cups mixed baby greens
12 long strands of chives
    (optional)

To make the Sesame Vinaigrette, place the garlic in the work bowl of a food processor fitted with a metal blade (or in a blender) and process until finely chopped. Add the vinegar, soy sauce, mustard, and salt and process until blended. Add the peanut oil (or canola oil) and sesame oil in a slow, steady stream and process until well blended. Set aside. (The vinaigrette can be made a day ahead. Transfer the vinaigrette to a covered container and refrigerate until 1 hour before serving. When ready to use, whisk the vinaigrette to blend and taste for seasoning.)

Combine the shrimp, mushrooms, and green onions in a medium bowl and lightly blend. Add just enough Sesame Vinaigrette to very lightly coat the salad components. (The Sesame Vinaigrette is very strongly flavored—a little goes a long way.)

To serve, make a bed of the mixed baby greens on each of four dinner plates. Arrange the shrimp salad on top of the greens, dividing evenly. Garnish each salad with long strands of fresh chives randomly scattered over the top, if desired.

For a simpler presentation, combine the salad ingredients in a large bowl. Add just enough Sesame Vinaigrette to make the lettuce leaves glisten.

EACH SERVING PROVIDES:

13g carbohydrates, 429 calories, 34g protein, 27g fat,

3g dietary fiber, 1249mg sodium, 222mg cholesterol

Tarragon Chicken Salad

Tarragon is an herb that adds a delightfully subtle licorice flavor to most foods. I particularly like the combination of a main course chicken salad dressed with a Tarragon Vinaigrette. Of course, feel free to substitute any of your favorite vinaigrettes for the one I have suggested.

4 SERVINGS

6 tablespoons chicken broth

3 tablespoons good-quality walnut oil

3 tablespoons sherry vinegar

1 tablespoon fresh tarragon leaves (or 1 teaspoon dried tarragon leaves)

1 tablespoon finely chopped fresh chives

1 clove garlic, finely chopped

½ tablespoon Dijon mustard

¼ teaspoon coarse salt

⅛ teaspoon freshly ground pepper

2 tablespoons extra virgin olive oil

4 skinless, boneless chicken breast halves (5 ounces each)

Salt and freshly ground pepper, to taste

6 cups mixed baby greens

4 ounces cooked greens beans, cooked until crisp-tender

To make the Tarragon Vinaigrette, place the chicken broth in a small saucepan over medium-high heat and bring to a boil. Cook for 5 to 7 minutes or until broth is reduced to 3 tablespoons. Set aside to cool to room temperature.

Combine the reduced chicken broth, walnut oil, 2 tablespoons of the sherry vinegar, tarragon, chives, garlic, mustard, salt, and pepper in a jar with a tight-fitting lid. Shake until well blended. (The vinaigrette can be made a day ahead. Refrigerate until 1 hour before serving. When ready to use, whisk the vinaigrette to blend and taste for seasoning.)

Heat a large skillet over medium-high heat for 2 minutes. Add the olive oil and swirl the pan to coat the bottom evenly. Season the chicken breasts with salt and pepper and place them in the skillet. Cook for 4 to 5 minutes on each side or until lightly brown. Add the remaining 1 tablespoon sherry vinegar and continue cooking until the liquid has evaporated.

Remove the chicken breasts to a cutting board and allow them to cool for 10 minutes. When cool, carve the chicken breasts into thin slices.

To serve, arrange a bed of the mixed baby greens on each of four dinner plates. Place overlapping slices of chicken on top of the greens and randomly distribute the green beans on top. Drizzle the Tarragon Vinaigrette over each serving.

EACH SERVING PROVIDES:

5g carbohydrates, 461 calories, 44g protein, 29g fat,
2g dietary fiber, 386mg sodium, 119mg cholesterol

* * * * * * * * *

GREEN WITH ENVY SALADS

A well-chosen salad is a healthy and flavorful addition to any meal. Fortunately, many traditional salad ingredients are low in carbohydrates, so the possibilities for filling your salad bowl with a savory treat that will fit your chosen diet plan are almost endless.

Asparagus and Walnut Salad

When you can't decide whether to serve a salad or a vegetable, this cold asparagus salad deliciously solves the dilemma. You will be surprised how wonderful walnuts and asparagus taste when combined in this delectable field of greens.

4 SERVINGS

1 pound asparagus spears, tough ends removed
6 cups mixed baby greens

1 recipe Walnut Vinaigrette (page 129)
¼ cup (or more) coarsely chopped walnuts

FILL a large bowl with ice water and set aside.
Bring water to a rolling boil in a large skillet. Add the asparagus and blanch for 1 minute. Transfer the asparagus to a colander to drain quickly. Immediately immerse in ice water. Drain. Pat dry with paper towels.

To serve, arrange a bed of mixed baby greens on each of four salad plates. Place the asparagus spears on the greens, dividing evenly among the servings. Drizzle Walnut Vinaigrette over the salad and garnish the top of each serving with walnuts.

EACH SERVING PROVIDES:
9g carbohydrates, 330 calories, 6g protein, 32g fat,
4g dietary fiber, 186mg sodium, 0mg cholesterol

(continues)

ABOUT ASPARAGUS

Asparagus adds color and a distinctive flavor to most foods. When buying asparagus in the spring, choose ones that are pencil thin. As the season progresses, the fatter ones will taste best. The stalks should be firm with tips that have tightly closed buds. Since asparagus begins to lose its sweetness as soon as it is cut, it is best to look for stems that appear to be freshly cut and not dried out.

Before cooking asparagus, hold on to both ends of each spear and gently snap. It will naturally break where it is tough and fibrous, leaving only the most tender portion of the vegetable.

Caesar Salad

The Caesar salad was invented in the 1920s by Caesar Cardini, the owner of an Italian restaurant in Tijuana, Mexico. This famous dish originally was known as the "aviator's salad," but Cardini later renamed it "Caesar's salad." This versatile dish is a wonderful complement to any dinner. It can be magically transformed into main course fare by simply adding grilled chicken strips, salmon, shrimp, or vegetables, or the thick and savory salad dressing can be served as a dip with an assortment of low-carbohydrate vegetables. It is too good to be true!

4 SERVINGS

1 clove garlic
4 anchovy fillets, drained
2 tablespoons fresh lemon juice
2 teaspoons Dijon mustard
1 egg yolk*
½ teaspoon freshly ground pepper
¼ teaspoon coarse salt

½ cup extra virgin olive oil
2 tablespoons (1 ounce) freshly grated Parmesan cheese
6 cups romaine lettuce, torn into generous bite-size pieces
2 tablespoons (1 ounce) shaved Parmesan cheese

To make the Caesar Dressing, place the garlic in the work bowl of a food processor fitted with a metal blade (or in a blender) and process until finely chopped. Add the anchovies and chop again. Add the lemon juice, mustard, egg yolk, pepper, and salt and blend well. Pour the olive oil through the feed tube in a slow, steady stream and mix until smooth. Add the grated cheese and process just to blend. (The dressing can be made a day ahead. Transfer it to a covered container and refrigerate until 1 hour before serving. When ready to use, whisk the dressing to blend, and taste for seasoning.)

(continues)

---

*If you are concerned about adding a raw yolk to the dressing, simply omit the egg.

To serve the salad, place the romaine lettuce in a large bowl and add just enough Caesar Dressing to coat the lettuce leaves; toss well. Arrange the salad on each of four salad plates and garnish each serving with shaved Parmesan cheese. The remaining Caesar Dressing can be refrigerated in a covered container for 1 to 2 days.

EACH SERVING PROVIDES:

4g carbohydrates, 322 calories, 6g protein, 32g fat,
2g dietary fiber, 453mg sodium, 61mg cholesterol

ABOUT ROMAINE LETTUCE

Romaine lettuce is named after the Greek island of Cos, where it originated. This lettuce has long, coarse green outer leaves while the whiter leaves in the center are the tastiest and crispiest.

Cauliflower (sans Potato) Salad

Why sans potatoes? This exceptional salad is made with all of the ingredients traditionally found in a potato salad. Since potatoes are high in carbohydrates, you can still indulge in this all-American favorite by substituting with cauliflower. The recipe can be doubled or tripled.

4 SERVINGS

2 pounds cauliflower (or 3 cups cauliflower florets)
½ cup (or more) mayonnaise
1 teaspoon white wine vinegar
1 teaspoon yellow mustard
¼ teaspoon coarse salt
3 hard-boiled eggs, chopped
⅓ cup diced red onion
1 red bell pepper, diced

PLACE a steamer in a large saucepan filled with about 2 inches of water. Bring the water to a boil over medium-high heat. Place the cauliflower in the steamer. Cover, and cook for 8 to 10 minutes or just until crisp-tender. Drain well. Set aside to cool to room temperature.

Combine the mayonnaise, white wine vinegar, mustard, and salt in a small bowl and blend well.

Combine the cauliflower, eggs, red onion, and red pepper in a large bowl and lightly blend. Add the mayonnaise mixture and blend until all the salad components are coated. Cover the bowl and refrigerate for several hours or overnight.

EACH SERVING PROVIDES:
15g carbohydrates, 321 calories, 9g protein, 26g fat,
7g dietary fiber, 410mg sodium, 160mg cholesterol

Greek Salad

Greek salad has evolved into much more than a simple salad. It is hearty enough to be served as a main course salad and yet can be served in smaller portions to accompany most Mediterranean dishes.

4 SERVINGS

3 tablespoons red wine vinegar
½ teaspoon coarse salt
¼ teaspoon Splenda or other artificial sweetener
⅛ teaspoon freshly ground pepper
¾ teaspoon dry mustard
¾ teaspoon dried oregano leaves
¼ teaspoon minced garlic clove
¼ teaspoon fresh lemon juice
½ cup extra virgin olive oil

6 cups romaine lettuce, broken into generous bite-size pieces
½ cup thinly sliced yellow onion
1 green bell pepper, seeds removed, cored, and thinly sliced
6 ounces feta cheese, crumbled
8 Greek olives (Kalamatas)
4 Greek peppers (pepperoncini)
~~8 anchovy fillets, drained and separated~~
~~4 hard-boiled eggs,~~ quartered
1 cucumber,

To make the Greek Vinaigrette, combine the vinegar, salt, Splenda, pepper, mustard, oregano, garlic, and lemon juice in the work bowl of a food processor fitted with a metal blade (or in a blender) and process until blended. Let the mixture sit for at least 15 minutes to allow the flavors to steep.

When ready, add the olive oil in a slow, steady stream and mix until smooth. Combine the lettuce, onion, green pepper, and cheese in a large salad bowl. Add enough Greek Vinaigrette to make the lettuce glisten; gently toss.

To serve, arrange the salad on each of four chilled salad plates and garnish each serving with the Greek olives, *feta* ~~anchovies~~, Greek peppers, ~~anchovies~~, and eggs, dividing evenly among the servings.

EACH SERVING PROVIDES:

11g carbohydrates, 510 calories, 16g protein, 45g fat, 3g dietary fiber, 1743mg sodium, 232mg cholesterol

Mixed Baby Greens with Blue Cheese and Walnuts

Mixed baby greens add a wonderful variety of colors and texture to this salad. The salad is equally delicious when made with fresh spinach.

4 SERVINGS

2 tablespoons white wine
   vinegar
1 tablespoon Dijon mustard
1 tablespoon fresh lemon juice
¼ teaspoon coarse salt
⅛ teaspoon freshly ground
   pepper

¼ cup canola oil
6 cups mixed baby greens
½ small red onion, thinly sliced
½ cup crumbled Maytag Blue
   Cheese or favorite blue
   cheese
¼ cup chopped walnuts

To make the White Wine Vinaigrette, whisk the vinegar, mustard, lemon juice, salt, and pepper in a small bowl until blended. Gradually whisk in the canola oil until well blended.

To serve, combine the mixed baby greens, red onion, cheese, and walnuts in a salad bowl. Add enough White Wine Vinaigrette to make the lettuce leaves glisten and gently toss. Season with salt and pepper, if desired.

EACH SERVING PROVIDES:
5g carbohydrates, 251 calories, 7g protein, 23g fat,
2g dietary fiber, 470mg sodium, 13mg cholesterol

ABOUT MIXED BABY GREENS

Mixed baby greens also are known as *mesclun* (French), *misticanza* (Italian), and spring greens. When this mixture of salad leaves and herbs is used in a salad, it provides a wonderful array of vivid colors, exotic flavors, and contrasting textures. Originally, these salad ingredients could only be obtained from the wild in Europe. Today, they are available in supermarkets by the pound or in cellophane bags.

Mixed Baby Greens, Endive, Roquefort, and Walnut Salad

The marriage of Roquefort cheese and walnuts combined with delicate greens results in a salad that achieves a five-star rating. So rich in flavor, it needs nothing more than pork or beef tenderloin to make it into a simple but elegant meal.

4 SERVINGS

6 cups mixed baby greens
1 endive, trimmed and cut into
  julienne strips
2 ounces Roquefort cheese,
  crumbled

¼ cup (or more) coarsely
  chopped walnuts
1 recipe Walnut Vinaigrette
  (page 129)
Edible flowers, for garnish

COMBINE the mixed baby greens, endive, cheese, and walnuts in a large bowl. Add enough Walnut Vinaigrette to make the leaves glisten.

To serve, arrange the salad on each of four salad plates, dividing evenly among the servings. Garnish with an edible flower, if desired.

EACH SERVING PROVIDES:

4g carbohydrates, 358 calories, 6g protein, 36g fat,
2g dietary fiber, 440mg sodium, 13mg cholesterol

ABOUT EDIBLE FLOWERS

. . . .

Edible flowers can add interest and color to most salads. They not only are decorative when used as a garnish but they also add a noticeable piquancy to a salad. The most widely available edible flowers are rose petals, calendula flowers, chrysanthemums, carnations, violets, and nasturtium flowers or leaves. These flowers can be found prewashed and free from harmful chemicals in the produce section of many supermarkets. Avoid any fresh flowers from the florist because they may be sprayed with chemicals.

Mixed Baby Greens with Goat Cheese

An easy-to-prepare salad that reaches company status when garnished with slices of goat cheese. If you don't have time to make your own raspberry vinaigrette, try one of the many commercial varieties available in most supermarkets.

4 SERVINGS

1 shallot
½ cup canola oil
2 tablespoons raspberry vinegar
1 tablespoon Dijon mustard
⅛ teaspoon coarse salt
⅛ teaspoon freshly ground
  pepper

6 cups mixed baby greens
4 slices goat cheese (such as
  Montrachet), cut ½-inch
  thick
Edible flowers, for garnish

To make the Raspberry Vinaigrette, place the shallot in the work bowl of a food processor fitted with a metal blade (or in a blender) and process until finely chopped. Add the oil, vinegar, mustard, salt, and pepper and process until well blended. (The vinaigrette can be made a day ahead. Transfer to a covered container and refrigerate until one hour before serving. When ready to use, whisk the vinaigrette to blend and taste for seasoning.)

Place the mixed baby greens in a salad bowl and add enough raspberry vinaigrette to make the lettuce leaves glisten; toss well.

To serve, arrange the salad on each of four salad plates and place a slice of cheese on top of the greens or off to the side. Garnish with an edible flower, if desired.

EACH SERVING PROVIDES:

4g carbohydrates, 312 calories, 5g protein, 32g fat,
2g dietary fiber, 240mg sodium, 11mg cholesterol

Mixed Baby Greens with Shallot Vinaigrette

During the holidays, I like to serve a simple green salad because it adds color and texture and nicely complements the other dishes. If you prefer not to use mixed baby greens, choose any of your other favorite low-carbohydrate greens.

4 SERVINGS

1 shallot
2 tablespoons red wine vinegar
1 tablespoon Dijon mustard
1 tablespoon chopped fresh
  parsley
¼ teaspoon coarse salt
⅛ teaspoon freshly ground
  pepper

⅛ teaspoon Splenda or other
  artificial sweetener
5 tablespoons extra virgin
  olive oil
6 cups mixed baby greens
Edible flowers, for garnish

To make the Shallot Vinaigrette, place the shallot in the work bowl of a food processor fitted with a metal blade (or in a blender) and process until finely chopped. Add the vinegar, mustard, parsley, salt, pepper, and Splenda and blend well. Add the olive oil in a slow, steady stream and process until well blended. (The vinaigrette can be made a day ahead. Transfer it to a covered container and refrigerate until 1 hour before serving. When ready to use, whisk the vinaigrette to blend and taste for seasoning.)

Place the mixed baby greens in a salad bowl and add enough Shallot Vinaigrette to make the lettuce leaves glisten; toss well.

To serve, arrange the salad on each of four salad plates and garnish each serving with an edible flower, if desired.

EACH SERVING PROVIDES:
4g carbohydrates, 179 calories, 2g protein, 18g fat,
2g dietary fiber, 234mg sodium, 0mg cholesterol

ABOUT SHALLOTS

Like garlic and onion, the shallot is a member of the lily family. It is milder in taste than onion and less pungent than garlic. The shallot is similar in size to a garlic bulb but can be identified by its brown papery skin and elongated bulb that is tapered at one end. Look for shallots that are plump, small, and firm. Be sure to avoid any that are dried out as they tend to have little flavor. Shallots can be found in the produce section of most supermarkets.

Mixed Baby Greens with Tarragon-Scented Vinaigrette

Dressing a simple salad of mixed baby greens with this sensational Tarragon-Scented Vinaigrette transforms it into a culinary delight.

4 SERVINGS

2 teaspoons chopped shallot
1 clove garlic
½ cup extra virgin olive oil
3 tablespoons tarragon vinegar
2 tablespoons chopped fresh
  parsley
1 teaspoon Dijon mustard
½ teaspoon coarse salt

¼ teaspoon Splenda or other
  artificial sweetener
¼ teaspoon freshly ground
  pepper
8 cups mixed baby greens
Edible flowers, for garnish

To make the Tarragon-Scented Vinaigrette, place the shallot and garlic in the work bowl of a food processor fitted with a metal blade (or in a blender) and process until finely chopped. Add the olive oil, vinegar, parsley, mustard, salt, Splenda, and pepper and process until smooth.

Place the mixed baby greens in a large salad bowl and add enough Tarragon-Scented Vinaigrette to make the leaves glisten. Toss well.

To serve, arrange the salad on each of four salad plates, dividing evenly among the servings. Garnish each serving with an edible flower, if desired.

EACH SERVING PROVIDES:
4g carbohydrates, 276 calories, 2g protein, 28g fat,
2g dietary fiber, 296mg sodium, 0mg cholesterol

Old-Fashioned Coleslaw

This recipe for coleslaw has been in my family for years. It is delicious with cabbage alone, but for a change of color and taste, you can add thinly sliced celery or red pepper. The cabbage can be thinly shredded in a food processor or, with patience, cut by hand.

4 SERVINGS

¾ cup mayonnaise
2 tablespoons Dijon mustard
1 tablespoon cider vinegar
1 teaspoon Splenda or other
    artificial sweetener
1 teaspoon celery seed

½ teaspoon celery salt
¼ teaspoon coarse salt
¼ teaspoon freshly ground
    pepper
1 pound cabbage, thinly grated

COMBINE all ingredients except the cabbage in a large bowl and blend well. Add the shredded cabbage and toss well. Taste for seasoning. The coleslaw can be served immediately or refrigerated, covered, for several hours or overnight.

EACH SERVING PROVIDES:
8g carbohydrates, 342 calories, 2g protein, 34g fat,
3g dietary fiber, 739mg sodium, 30mg cholesterol

Romaine Salad with Romano Cheese

This salad is similar in taste and appearance to the classic Caesar Salad (page 139), but there are a variety of ingredients in this vinaigrette that are not traditionally found in the original. As far as I am concerned, you can never have enough Caesar salad recipes.

4 SERVINGS

3 tablespoons fresh lemon juice

1 egg*

½ teaspoon coarse salt

½ teaspoon freshly ground
   pepper

¼ teaspoon dried oregano
   leaves

¼ teaspoon ground turmeric

⅛ teaspoon dried mint leaves

½ cup extra virgin olive oil

6 cups romaine lettuce, torn
   into generous bite-size pieces

½ cup (or more) freshly grated
   Romano cheese

To make the Caesar II Dressing, place the lemon juice, egg, salt, pepper, oregano, turmeric, and mint in the work bowl of a food processor fitted with a metal blade (or in a blender) and process until blended. Add the olive oil in a slow, steady stream and mix until smooth. (The dressing can be made a day ahead. Transfer it to a covered container and refrigerate until 1 hour before serving. When ready to use, whisk the dressing to blend and taste for seasoning.)

To serve, place the lettuce and cheese in a large bowl and toss. Add just enough Caesar II Dressing to coat the lettuce leaves; toss well. Arrange the salad on each of four salad plates, dividing evenly among the servings.

EACH SERVING PROVIDES:
4g carbohydrates, 333 calories, 7g protein, 33g fat,
2g dietary fiber, 406mg sodium, 60mg cholesterol

*If you are concerned about adding a raw egg, simply omit the egg.

Spinach Salad with Bacon

This spinach salad is one of my favorites to serve with flank steak or other beef recipes. It also can be enjoyed as a main dish luncheon salad.

6 SERVINGS

½ cup canola oil
¼ cup garlic red wine vinegar
2 tablespoons dry white wine
2 teaspoons soy sauce
1 teaspoon dry mustard
½ teaspoon curry powder
½ teaspoon coarse salt

½ teaspoon freshly ground pepper
1 package (10 ounces) pre-washed fresh baby spinach
5 slices bacon, cooked, drained, and crumbled
2 hard-boiled eggs, finely chopped

To prepare the Garlic Red Wine Vinaigrette, combine the oil, vinegar, wine, soy sauce, mustard, curry powder, salt, and pepper in the work bowl of a food processor fitted with a metal blade (or in a blender) and process until smooth. The vinaigrette also can be prepared in a jar with a tight-fitting lid. Add the ingredients to the jar and shake until well blended.

To serve, place the spinach in a large bowl and add enough Garlic Red Wine Vinaigrette to make the spinach leaves glisten. Divide the salad on each of six salad plates and garnish each serving with bacon and eggs. Alternatively, place the spinach, eggs, and bacon in a salad bowl. Add the vinaigrette and gently toss.

EACH SERVING PROVIDES:
2g carbohydrates, 231 calories, 5g protein, 23g fat,
1g dietary fiber, 413mg sodium, 67mg cholesterol

Spinach Salad with Blue Cheese Vinaigrette

Dressing a spinach salad with the savory Blue Cheese Vinaigrette provides just the right balance in flavors. You will adore it!

6 SERVINGS

6 tablespoons extra virgin olive oil

¼ cup (1½ ounces) Maytag Blue Cheese or favorite blue cheese, crumbled

3 tablespoons balsamic vinegar

1½ tablespoons soy sauce

¼ teaspoon coarse salt

¼ teaspoon freshly ground pepper

6 cups prewashed spinach

1 red bell pepper, cut into julienne strips

2 green onions, thinly sliced

To make the Blue Cheese Vinaigrette, combine the olive oil, cheese, vinegar, soy sauce, salt, and pepper in a jar with a tight-fitting lid and shake until well blended. (The vinaigrette can be made a day ahead. Refrigerate until 1 hour before serving. When ready to use, whisk the vinaigrette to blend and taste for seasoning.)

To make the salad, place the spinach, red pepper, and green onions in a salad bowl. Add enough Blue Cheese Vinaigrette to coat the salad ingredients; gently toss. To serve, arrange the salad on each of six salad plates, dividing evenly among the servings.

EACH SERVING PROVIDES:
4g carbohydrates, 166 calories, 3g protein, 16g fat,
1g dietary fiber, 440mg sodium, 4mg cholesterol

ABOUT SPINACH

Spinach has dark green arrow-shaped leaves. It is one of the most versatile of salad ingredients because of its complementary distinctive taste, wonderful texture, and rich color. Spinach is quite perishable, however. It will only stay fresh for 2 to 3 days, so it is best to store it with care and use it as soon as possible.

When choosing spinach, look for baby spinach or spinach with crisp, dark green leaves. Remove any blackened leaves and store the remaining spinach in a resealable plastic bag in the refrigerator. It is also very important to wash spinach well just before using it in a salad because it is a low-lying plant that collects sand and soil particles while growing. If you buy prewashed spinach, which is widely available in cellophane bags, open the bag and remove any blackened leaves. Reseal the bag and store it in the refrigerator until you are ready to prepare your salad.

Spinach Salad with Maytag Blue Cheese

You will be tempted to serve this green, red, and white salad during the festive holidays. Its robust flavor nicely complements beef or poultry.

6 SERVINGS

6 cups prewashed spinach
3 cups Boston lettuce, torn into
  generous bite-size pieces
3 green onions, thinly sliced
3 ounces Maytag Blue Cheese
  or favorite blue cheese,
  crumbled

1 recipe Balsamic Vinaigrette
  (page 118)
1 red pepper, thinly sliced

COMBINE the spinach, lettuce, green onions, and cheese in a large bowl. Add enough Balsamic Vinaigrette to make the leaves glisten. To serve, arrange the salad on each of six salad plates. Randomly distribute the red pepper strips over each serving.

EACH SERVING PROVIDES:
5g carbohydrates, 242 calories, 5g protein, 23g fat,
2g dietary fiber, 422mg sodium, 11mg cholesterol

chapter seven

MASTERFUL
MAIN COURSES

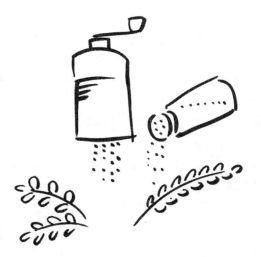

MAIN COURSES

Rise and Shine

Chiles Rellenos Casserole

Crab Frittata

Crab and Shrimp Scrambled
  Eggs

Eggs and Italian Sausage
  Casserole

Monterey Jack Cheese Quiche

Mushroom Omelet

Quiche Lorraine

Scrambled Eggs with Smoked
  Salmon

Smoked Salmon Omelet

Southwestern Tofu Scramble

Wild Mushroom and Green
  Onion Omelet

Hot and Spicy

Better Than Hot Pork Tenderloin

Chipotle Marinated Flank Steak

Creole Shrimp

Jamaican Pork Tenderloin

Lamb Vindaloo

Pacific Rim Pork Tenderloin

Peppered Shrimp

Sesame-Coated Salmon with
  Wasabi Sauce

Southwestern Shrimp with
  Creamy Chipotle Sauce

On the Grill

Butterflied Leg of Lamb

Cornish Hens with Jerk Rub

Greek Chicken

Grilled Mediterranean Lemon
  Chicken

Grilled Thai Shrimp with
  Dipping Sauce

Lemon and Tarragon Marinated
  Salmon

Savory Rubbed Baby Back Ribs

Shish Kebab

Southwestern Rubbed Flank
  Steak

Swordfish with Olive and Red
  Pepper Relish

Tandoori Chicken

Tex-Mex Flank Steak with
  Gazpacho Salsa

Tuna Fajitas

Exotic Flavors

Asian Rubbed Salmon

Caribbean Rubbed Flank Steak

Cornish Hens with Thai Rub
Cuban Pork Loin Roast
Lemongrass Marinated Whole
    Chicken
Mediterranean Turkey Patties
Moroccan Chicken with Sliced
    Almonds
New Delhi Turkey Meatloaf
Pacific Rim Marinated Salmon
Veal Piccata

In the Main
Beef Tenderloin with
    Mushroom Sauce
Cornish Hens with Lemon
    Glaze
Curried Mustard-Coated
    Flank Steak
Lemon Chicken
Maytag Blue Cheese Stuffed
    Pork Chops
Mustard-Coated Leg of Lamb
Original Joe's Special

Poached Salmon with Mustard
    Dill Sauce
Pork Chops with Red Peppers
Salmon Glazed with Dill
    Butter
Salmon with Saffron
    Vinaigrette
Spicy Chicken Thighs
Spicy Lamb Chops

Strictly Vegetarian
Curried Tempeh with Spinach
Indonesian Tempeh
Orange-Scented Tofu Stir-Fry
Portobello Eggplant Pizzas
Roasted Vegetable Torte with
    Harissa Vinaigrette
Spicy Tofu
Spinach and Ricotta Tart
Thai Marinated Portobello
    Mushrooms
Tofu Curry

THE MAIN COURSE IS the most eagerly anticipated culinary experience of every meal. Who doesn't relish the thought of savoring a quiche studded with bacon and cheese first thing in the morning, indulging in an artful main course salad at midday, or dining on a delicately spiced poultry ensemble in the evening? These low-carbohydrate centerpieces, richly flavored and satisfying, clearly refute the notion that this way of dining need ever be boring.

At first glance, the selection of foods allowed on a low-carbohydrate diet may appear to be limited in scope. However, most of the foods can be magically transformed into a variety of temptingly delicious offerings. A chicken breast is an example of how versatile a main course staple can be. Simply varying the way it is prepared can make the difference between a gourmet delight and a ho-hum experience. While baked chicken breast will always remain a scrumptious treat, it easily can be elevated to the next level of flavor intensity by infusing it with the smoky aroma of your patio grill. In addition to grilling and baking, you also can stir-fry, poach, sauté, or broil it to create a variety of taste sensations.

But let's not stop here. How you prepare the chicken breast is only a prelude to the almost unlimited number of ways that you can vary its taste. For example, before cooking a chicken breast, its flavors can be greatly enhanced by simply adding such ingredients as herbs and spices, zesty marinades, or a savory rub. Each of these flavoring ingredients will imbue it with a signature taste that will linger long after the last bite. But the humble chicken breast's journey to gourmet status is not finished yet. Sautéed, it can become an elegant feast when nestled in a delectable sauce spooned on to a plate or over the chicken breast. That same chicken breast can be served on a bed of zucchini pasta, topped with a zesty salsa, or made into a main course salad—the endless combinations are limited only by your imagination. By simply varying the way you prepare, season, or adorn a chicken breast, or other component of a main course meal, you will be able to create a bounty of mealtime offerings for your family and friends.

As you read through the recipes, you will note that some of them do not suggest using low-fat or nonfat ingredients. As previously mentioned, such substitutions are always welcome, especially if you find that you are not losing weight as quickly as you would like or are concerned about the health risks of certain foods. Likewise, if you prefer a vegetarian menu, many of the main courses made with poultry or meat, for example, can be substituted with your favorite soybean product. I have identified several such recipes by noting a Vegetarian Variation at the end of each. With a little imagination, you can adapt other recipes to your vegetarian tastes as well.

I hope you will share in my enthusiasm for the infinite number of ways low-carbohydrate dieting can be exciting and rewarding. With so many possibilities for creating palate-pleasing delights, you will find it easy to confirm your commitment to this way of dining.

RISE AND SHINE

Starting the day off eating a nutritious breakfast is one way of supplying yourself with a healthy portion of the daily recommended levels of essential nutrients. Not only are these rise-and-shine delights a healthy start, they also can be savored as a midday snack.

Chiles Rellenos Casserole

Enjoying this zesty egg dish first thing in the morning is the perfect way to start the day with a bang. Leftovers can be kept refrigerated and served the next day.

6 SERVINGS

9 large eggs
¼ cup whipping cream
½ cup shredded Monterey Jack cheese
½ cup shredded sharp Cheddar cheese
½ cup diced red bell pepper
1 can (4 ounces) chopped green chilies

1 tablespoon minced yellow onion
¼ teaspoon coarse salt
⅛ teaspoon freshly ground pepper
1 to 2 dashes Tabasco sauce or favorite hot pepper sauce

PREHEAT oven to 350 degrees F. Lightly coat a 1½- to 2-quart baking dish with a nonstick vegetable spray. Set aside.

Combine the eggs and whipping cream in a medium bowl and whisk until well blended. Add the rest of the ingredients and blend well. Pour the mixture into the prepared baking dish. Bake for 40 minutes or until set in the center. Cool at least 10 minutes before serving.

EACH SERVING PROVIDES:

3g carbohydrates, 226 calories, 14g protein, 17g fat,
1g dietary fiber, 356mg sodium, 351mg cholesterol

Crab Frittata

The frittata is basically an Italian omelet. You will be delighted to find that this spicy frittata is exceptionally versatile. It can be served as the main course of any meal or enjoyed as a snack, and it remains equally delicious whether it is served warm or cold. If you favor shrimp over crab, feel free to use it instead.

4 SERVINGS

6 large eggs
2 tablespoons 2 percent milk
½ teaspoon coarse salt
½ teaspoon freshly ground
  pepper
2 cans (6 ounces each) lump
  crabmeat, drained

2 tablespoons extra virgin
  olive oil
3 green onions, thinly sliced
1 clove garlic, minced

PREHEAT oven to 400 degrees F. Combine the eggs, milk, salt, and pepper in a medium bowl and whisk until well blended. Add the crabmeat and blend.

Heat a large nonstick, ovenproof skillet over medium-high heat for 1 minute. Add the olive oil and swirl the pan to coat the bottom evenly. Add the green onions and garlic and sauté for 1 minute, stirring frequently. Add the egg mixture and lightly blend. Cook for 2 to 3 minutes or just until the bottom of the frittata has set.

Place the skillet in the oven and bake for 10 minutes or until the eggs are set.

Remove the skillet from the oven and invert the frittata onto a plate. Place another plate on top of the frittata and invert again so the frittata is right side up.

EACH SERVING PROVIDES:

2g carbohydrates, 266 calories, 27g protein, 16g fat,

0g dietary fiber, 618mg sodium, 395mg cholesterol

Crab and Shrimp Scrambled Eggs

Start the morning with this hearty scrambled egg and seafood composition. In fact, it is so satisfying you can serve it for lunch, too. This recipe easily can be doubled.

4 SERVINGS

6 eggs
6 tablespoons 2 percent milk
1 tablespoon chopped fresh
 chives
½ teaspoon seasoned salt
½ teaspoon coarse salt
⅛ teaspoon freshly ground
 pepper

2 to 3 (or more) drops Tabasco
 sauce or favorite hot pepper
 sauce
1 can (6 ounces) lump crabmeat, drained
1 can (4 ounces) medium-size
 shrimp, drained
2 tablespoons butter
Chives, for garnish (optional)

COMBINE the eggs, milk, chives, seasoned salt, salt, pepper, and Tabasco sauce in a medium bowl and whisk until well blended. Add the crabmeat and shrimp and blend.

Melt the butter in a large nonstick skillet over medium heat. Pour the egg mixture into the skillet and cook for 4 to 6 minutes or until the eggs have almost set, gently lifting the edges with a spatula and tilting the pan so the uncooked portion flows underneath.

To serve, divide the crab and shrimp scrambled eggs on each of four dinner plates. Garnish each serving with chives, if desired.

EACH SERVING PROVIDES:

2g carbohydrates, 251 calories, 26g protein, 15g fat,
0g dietary fiber, 706mg sodium, 423mg cholesterol

Eggs and Italian Sausage Casserole

This savory casserole is as Italian and spirited as an Alfa Romeo, and almost as fast. It can be assembled the night before and freshly baked first thing in the morning. The recipe can be halved also— just use a smaller baking dish.

8 SERVINGS

¾ cup sour cream
1 teaspoon coarse salt
½ teaspoon paprika
½ teaspoon dry mustard
¾ pound shredded sharp
    Cheddar cheese

1 pound sweet (or hot) Italian
    sausage, cooked and
    crumbled
8 eggs

PREHEAT oven to 325 degrees F. Lightly coat a 1½-quart baking dish with a nonstick vegetable spray and set aside.

Combine the sour cream, salt, paprika, and mustard in a small bowl and blend well.

Spread half the Cheddar cheese on the bottom of the prepared baking dish. Spoon dollops of half the sour cream mixture over the cheese. Distribute all the sausage over the sour cream and randomly break whole eggs over the sausage. Spoon dollops of the remaining sour cream over the eggs and cover with the remaining cheese. Bake for 25 to 30 minutes or until the eggs are set.

EACH SERVING PROVIDES:

2g carbohydrates, 386 calories, 23g protein, 30g fat,
0g dietary fiber, 840mg sodium, 298mg cholesterol

Monterey Jack Cheese Quiche

I cannot think of a more delightful way to start the day than sitting down to a breakfast consisting of this savory quiche. In fact, it is so satisfying you may want to consider it for lunch or even as a light dinner.

8 SERVINGS

1 tablespoon extra virgin
   olive oil
1 cup thinly sliced yellow onion
5 eggs
8 ounces shredded Monterey
   Jack cheese

8 ounces cottage cheese
2 tablespoons melted butter
1 tablespoon caraway seeds
½ teaspoon coarse salt
¼ teaspoon freshly ground
   pepper

PREHEAT oven to 400 degrees F. Lightly coat a 9-inch quiche or pie pan with a nonstick vegetable spray and set aside.

Heat a medium nonstick skillet over medium heat for 1 minute. Add the olive oil and swirl the pan to coat the bottom evenly. Add the onion and sauté for 10 minutes, stirring occasionally.

Whisk the eggs in a medium bowl until well blended. Add the sautéed onions and the rest of the ingredients and blend well.

Pour the mixture into the prepared pan. Bake for 15 minutes.

Reduce oven temperature to 350 degrees F. Bake for 30 to 35 minutes or until set in the center and golden brown on top. Cool at least 10 minutes before serving.

EACH SERVING PROVIDES:
3g carbohydrates, 232 calories, 15g protein, 18g fat,
1g dietary fiber, 425mg sodium, 170mg cholesterol

Mushroom Omelet

This omelet is a prime example of how a few basic ingredients can combine to make simply delicious breakfast fare.

2 SERVINGS

4 eggs, lightly beaten
¼ teaspoon coarse salt
¼ teaspoon freshly ground pepper
2 tablespoons extra virgin olive oil

6 tablespoons chopped yellow onion
4 ounces fresh button mushrooms, thinly sliced
⅔ cup cottage cheese
Chives, for garnish (optional)

COMBINE the eggs, salt, and pepper in a small bowl and whisk until well blended. Set aside.

Heat a large nonstick skillet over medium heat for 2 minutes. Add the olive oil and swirl the pan to coat the bottom evenly. Add the onion and mushrooms and sauté for 4 minutes, stirring occasionally. Transfer the onion mixture to a medium bowl and add the cottage cheese; blend well.

Add the egg mixture to the same skillet and cook for 1 to 2 minutes or until almost set, gently lifting the edges with a spatula and tilting the pan so the uncooked portion flows underneath. Spoon the cottage cheese mixture on the lower half of the omelet. Slightly raise the skillet and use a fork to gently fold the top half over the filling.

To serve, divide the omelet into two servings. Place each one on a dinner plate and garnish with long strands of chives, if desired.

EACH SERVING PROVIDES:
8g carbohydrates, 373 calories, 23g protein, 27g fat,
1g dietary fiber, 648mg sodium, 435mg cholesterol

Quiche Lorraine

The ever-popular quiche Lorraine remains a favorite egg dish to enjoy at breakfast. As this quiche is very rich, it is also ideal fare to serve for lunch or a light dinner. Any leftovers can be refrigerated and served the following morning.

12 SERVINGS

2 tablespoons butter
½ cup chopped yellow onion
1 cup sliced fresh button mushrooms
2 eggs
2 egg yolks
1½ cups half-and-half
2 tablespoons sour cream

½ pound bacon, cooked crisp, drained, and crumbled
¼ pound (1 cup) shredded Swiss cheese
1 teaspoon Dijon mustard
½ teaspoon coarse salt
¼ teaspoon freshly ground pepper
⅛ teaspoon cayenne pepper

PREHEAT oven to 350 degrees F. Lightly coat a quiche pan or a 1½-quart baking dish with a nonstick vegetable spray. Set aside.

Melt the butter in a medium skillet over medium heat. Add the onion and sauté for 3 minutes, stirring occasionally. Add the mushrooms and cook for 3 minutes or until softened, stirring occasionally. Set aside.

Combine the eggs, egg yolks, half-and-half, and sour cream in a medium bowl and whisk until well blended. Add the cooked onion mixture and the rest of the ingredients and blend well. Pour the mixture into the prepared pan. Bake for 40 to 45 minutes or until set in the center and golden brown on top. Cool at least 10 minutes before serving.

EACH SERVING PROVIDES:

2g carbohydrates, 161 calories, 8g protein, 13g fat,
0g dietary fiber, 242mg sodium, 107mg cholesterol

Scrambled Eggs with Smoked Salmon

What a delightful way to start the morning! Not only is this egg creation delicious but its sunny appearance is very visually appealing. The recipe can easily be doubled.

4 SERVINGS

2 tablespoons extra virgin
  olive oil
1 tablespoon butter
½ cup chopped yellow onion
8 eggs
3 tablespoons 2 percent milk
3 tablespoons chopped fresh
  chives

¼ teaspoon coarse salt
¼ teaspoon freshly ground
  pepper
6 ounces smoked salmon (lox),
  cut into thin strips
1 tablespoon chopped fresh
  chives (optional)

HEAT the olive oil and butter in a large nonstick skillet over medium heat until the butter melts. Add the onion and sauté for 10 to 15 minutes or until golden.

Combine the eggs, milk, chives, salt, and pepper in a medium bowl and whisk until well blended. Pour the egg mixture into the skillet and cook for 4 minutes or until the eggs have almost set, stirring occasionally. Add the salmon and cook for about 1 minute or until the eggs are cooked but still moist.

To serve, divide the scrambled eggs on each of four dinner plates. Garnish each serving with chives, if desired.

EACH SERVING PROVIDES:

4g carbohydrates, 301 calories, 21g protein, 22g fat,
0g dietary fiber, 1101mg sodium, 443mg cholesterol

Smoked Salmon Omelet

A friend gave me this recipe, which has been a family favorite for years. My husband usually has enough time to take two bites of his breakfast, but when I serve him this delicious creation, he cleans the plate. I prefer to make two big omelets and cut each into three portions, but it can also be made into six individual servings.

6 SERVINGS

12 eggs
1 teaspoon coarse salt
½ teaspoon freshly ground
 pepper
2 tablespoons extra virgin
 olive oil

6 ounces smoked salmon (lox),
 cut into thin strips
¼ cup thinly sliced green onion
½ cup diced cream cheese, at
 room temperature
Chopped chives or capers, for
 garnish (optional)

COMBINE the eggs, salt, and pepper in a medium bowl and whisk until well blended.

Heat a large nonstick skillet over medium heat for 2 minutes. Add half the olive oil and swirl the pan to coat the bottom evenly. Pour half the eggs into the skillet and cook until almost set, gently lifting the edges with a spatula and tilting the pan so the uncooked portion flows underneath. Arrange half the salmon, green onion, and cream cheese on the lower half of the omelet. Slightly raise the skillet and use a fork to gently fold the top half over the filling. Heat for 1 to 2 minutes to allow the cream cheese to melt. Slide the omelet onto a large plate. Repeat with the remaining olive oil, eggs, salmon, green onion, and cream cheese to make another omelet.

To serve, divide each omelet into three servings. Place each one on a dinner plate and garnish each serving with chopped chives or capers, if desired.

EACH SERVING PROVIDES:

2g carbohydrates, 293 calories, 19g protein, 23g fat,
0g dietary fiber, 1065mg sodium, 453mg cholesterol

Southwestern Tofu Scramble

This hot and spicy tofu dish not only tastes good but it is also good for you! If the diet plan you are following allows it, serve it topped with salsa and cubed avocado.

4 SERVINGS

1 package (16 ounces) extra firm tofu
½ tablespoon extra virgin olive oil
¼ cup diced and seeded tomato
1 can (4 ounces) chopped green chilies
¼ teaspoon coarse salt

¼ teaspoon freshly ground pepper
⅛ teaspoon cayenne pepper
4 ounces Monterey Jack cheese, diced
2 tablespoons coarsely chopped fresh cilantro leaves

PLACE the tofu on a double thickness of paper towels and blot dry. Dice and set aside.

Place a large nonstick skillet over medium heat for 2 minutes. Add the olive oil and swirl the pan to coat the bottom evenly. Add the tomato, chilies, salt, pepper, and cayenne and sauté for 3 minutes, stirring occasionally. Add the tofu and cheese and cook over medium-high heat for 5 minutes, stirring frequently. Remove the skillet from the heat. Add the cilantro and lightly blend.

EACH SERVING PROVIDES:
4g carbohydrates, 188 calories, 15g protein, 13g fat,
1g dietary fiber, 384mg sodium, 25mg cholesterol

Wild Mushroom and Green Onion Omelet

You will go "wild" over this delectable omelet. It is a delightful way to start the morning but is also hearty enough to be served as a light lunch. If you prefer the taste of button mushrooms, simply substitute them for the wild ones.

6 SERVINGS

2 tablespoons extra virgin olive oil

1 pound mixed fresh wild mushrooms (such as morels, creminis, and chanterelles), thinly sliced

4 green onions, thinly sliced

2 cloves garlic, minced

1 tablespoon red wine vinegar

8 eggs

½ teaspoon coarse salt

½ teaspoon freshly ground pepper

¼ cup chopped fresh parsley or chives, for garnish

HEAT a large nonstick skillet over medium-low heat for 2 minutes. Add the olive oil and swirl the pan to coat the bottom evenly. Add the mushrooms, green onions, garlic, and red wine vinegar and cook for 10 minutes, stirring occasionally.

Combine the eggs, salt, and pepper in a small bowl and whisk until well blended. Pour the egg mixture over the mushroom mixture and cook for 5 to 10 minutes or until the eggs are set, gently lifting the edges with a spatula and tilting the pan so the uncooked portion flows underneath.

To serve, divide the omelet into six servings. Place each one on a dinner plate and garnish with parsley or chives, if desired.

EACH SERVING PROVIDES:

4g carbohydrates, 170 calories, 12g protein, 11g fat, 2g dietary fiber, 271mg sodium, 283mg cholesterol

HOT AND SPICY

A meal that is low in carbohydrates doesn't have to be low in taste and excitement. If your preferred tastes are Caribbean, Creole, or South of the Border, you'll find examples of what you like with a pleasing kick in this section.

Better Than Hot Pork Tenderloin

If you crave hot food, this pork tenderloin is destined to become a favorite. Sriracha hot chili sauce imparts enough heat to the pork so that you're not likely to forget it! I would suggest that you double the recipe so you can use the leftover pork in the Pork Tenderloin and Goat Cheese Salad (page 129)—it is a red-hot combination. Serve with Zucchini Matchsticks (page 314).

4 SERVINGS

1 tablespoon canola oil
1 tablespoon (or less) Sriracha hot chili sauce or favorite hot pepper sauce
1 tablespoon Splenda or other artificial sweetener
1 tablespoon soy sauce
1 tablespoon minced fresh ginger
2 teaspoons chopped green onion
1 teaspoon Asian sesame oil
1 clove garlic, minced
1 pork tenderloin (1½ pounds)

To make the Fiery Marinade, combine all the ingredients except for the pork in a large resealable plastic bag and blend well. Add the pork tenderloin and turn to coat all over. Seal the bag, and refrigerate for several hours or overnight, turning the pork at least once.

Preheat oven to 325 degrees F. Lightly coat a shallow pan with a nonstick vegetable spray.

Remove the pork tenderloin from the marinade (reserve the marinade). Place the pork in the prepared pan. Bake for 45 to 55 minutes or until a meat thermometer registers 150 to 155 degrees F, occasionally basting the pork with the reserved marinade. Transfer the pork to a carving board and cover loosely with foil. Cool at least 10 minutes before carving it into thin slices.

(continues)

To serve, place overlapping slices of pork on each of four dinner plates, dividing evenly among the servings.

EACH SERVING PROVIDES:

1g carbohydrates, 257 calories, 36g protein, 11g fat,
0g dietary fiber, 330mg sodium, 101mg cholesterol

ABOUT PORK

Pork is being bred leaner today, making it a healthy alternative to other meats. When shopping for pork, look for meats with a pale pink color, which indicates that the pork came from a younger animal. I like to cook pork until a meat thermometer inserted into the thickest part of the meat registers 155 degrees F. At this temperature, you can be certain that the meat is safely cooked but is still tender and juicy.

To freeze pork, label and date a freezer bag and place the pork in it. It will keep in the freezer for two to three months.

Chipotle Marinated Flank Steak

Chipotles really heat up the marinade, and, along with the heat, these fiery peppers impart a fragrant, smoky flavor. I have used this marinade on chicken and pork as well.

For a real showstopper meal, top the flank steak with Gazpacho Salsa (page 214). Serve with Green Beans with Garlic and Red Pepper Flakes (page 296).

4 SERVINGS

½ cup fresh orange juice
2 chipotle chilies in adobo
  sauce, minced*
1 clove garlic, minced
1 tablespoon extra virgin
  olive oil
1 tablespoon red wine vinegar

1 teaspoon dried oregano leaves
½ teaspoon ground cumin
½ teaspoon coarse salt
½ teaspoon freshly ground
  pepper
1 flank steak (1½ pounds),
  pierced all over with a fork

To make the Chipotle Marinade, combine all the ingredients except the steak in a large resealable plastic bag and blend well. Add the flank steak and turn to coat all over. Seal the bag, and refrigerate for several hours or overnight, turning the steak at least once.

Lightly coat a broiler pan with a nonstick vegetable spray.

Remove the flank steak from the marinade (discard the marinade). Place the steak on the pan and put under a preheated broiler, 4 to 5 inches from the heat source, for 4 to 5 minutes on each side or until a meat thermometer registers 145 degrees F. Carve the flank steak across the grain into very thin diagonal slices. To serve, place overlapping slices of steak on each end of four dinner plates, dividing evenly among the servings.

(continues)

---

*Chipotles in Adobo sauce can be found in cans in the Mexican section of most supermarkets.

VARIATION: To grill the flank steak, place it on a grill coated with a nonstick vegetable spray over medium-hot coals. Sear the steak for 1 minute on each side. Cover the grill and cook for 5 to 6 minutes on each side.

EACH SERVING PROVIDES:

5g carbohydrates, 326 calories, 36g protein, 17g fat,

1g dietary fiber, 460mg sodium, 88mg cholesterol

Creole Shrimp

Creole cooking and southern Louisiana are forever bound to each other. The Creoles were wealthy European aristocrats lured by the Spanish to establish New Orleans in the 1690s. When they came to the New World, the Creoles also brought their chefs and cooks from France and Spain who combined their knowledge of the grand cuisine of Europe with the local foodstuffs and, in the end, created "Creole" cooking.

4 SERVINGS

3 tablespoons extra virgin olive oil

2 tablespoons (or less) Creole seasoning

2 tablespoons fresh lemon juice

2 tablespoons chopped fresh parsley

1 tablespoon Splenda or other artificial sweetener

1 tablespoon soy sauce

⅛ teaspoon (or less) cayenne pepper

1½ pounds fresh large raw shrimp, peeled and deveined

To make the Creole Marinade, combine all the ingredients except the shrimp in a large resealable plastic bag and blend well. Add the shrimp and turn to coat all over. Seal the bag, and refrigerate for several hours or overnight, turning the shrimp at least once.

Preheat oven to 450 degrees F. Lightly coat a rimmed baking sheet with a nonstick vegetable spray.

Remove the shrimp from the marinade (discard the marinade). Place the shrimp in a single layer on the prepared baking sheet. Bake for 6 to 8 minutes or until the shrimp are no longer pink.

EACH SERVING PROVIDES:

2g carbohydrates, 269 calories, 36g protein, 12g fat,
0g dietary fiber, 638mg sodium, 332mg cholesterol

(continues)

ABOUT SHRIMP

Shrimp, as well as other seafood, are highly perishable. For this reason, it is very important to select fresh, high-quality shrimp, to store them properly, and to use them as quickly as possible.

When buying shrimp in their shells, look for shiny, tight-fitting shells. If the shrimp are already shelled, make sure they are dry and firm. Avoid any shrimp with black discoloration along the head or belly, as well as shrimp that have an ammonia odor. It is always best to buy your seafood the day you plan to use it and also to store it in the coldest part of the refrigerator until needed.

Jamaican Pork Tenderloin

The rise in popularity of Caribbean cooking has been spectacular in recent years. This cuisine features a wide variety of unique and interesting spices and ingredients that result in wonderfully spicy and flavorful dishes. Jamaican Pork Tenderloin typifies this culinary trend. The marinade imbues pork with a fabulous flavor but also makes it very hot! To make this dish less hot, reduce the suggested amount of hot pepper sauce. Also, by doubling the marinade ingredients, half of it can be reserved to make into a warm sauce to spoon over each serving. Serve with Green Beans and Red Pepper (page 292).

6 SERVINGS

½ cup minced yellow onion
¼ cup pickled jalapeño peppers
2 tablespoons soy sauce
2 tablespoons cold water
1 tablespoon extra virgin
    olive oil
1 large clove garlic, minced
1 teaspoon ground allspice
1 teaspoon freshly ground
    pepper

½ teaspoon ground cinnamon
½ teaspoon ground nutmeg
½ teaspoon dried thyme leaves
⅛ teaspoon coarse salt
⅛ teaspoon hot pepper sauce
1 pork tenderloin (2¼ pounds)
Coarsely chopped cilantro, for
    garnish (optional)

To make the Jamaican Marinade, combine all the ingredients except for the pork in a large resealable plastic bag and blend well. Place the pork tenderloin in the marinade and turn to coat both sides. Seal the bag, and refrigerate for several hours or overnight.

Preheat oven to 325 degrees F. Lightly coat a shallow pan with a nonstick vegetable spray.

(continues)

Remove the pork tenderloin from the marinade (reserve the marinade). Place the pork in the prepared pan. Bake for 45 to 55 minutes or until a meat thermometer registers 150 to 155 degrees F, occasionally basting the pork with the reserved marinade. Transfer the pork to a carving board and cover loosely with foil. Cool at least 10 minutes before carving it into thin slices.

To serve, place the overlapping slices of pork on each of six dinner plates, dividing evenly among the servings. Garnish each serving with coarsely chopped cilantro, if desired.

EACH SERVING PROVIDES:

5g carbohydrates, 252 calories, 37g protein, 9g fat,
1g dietary fiber, 598mg sodium, 101mg cholesterol

Lamb Vindaloo

This wonderful Indian dish illustrates how much piquancy can be created when a wide variety of spices are combined with the distinctive flavor of lamb. Vindaloos tend to be very hot, but you can make them a bit milder by decreasing the amount of cayenne pepper called for in the recipe or even by substituting coconut milk for the chicken broth. Please don't let the number of ingredients frighten you away from preparing this dish. If you have each one in front of you before starting the marinade, you will discover how quick it is to prepare.

4 SERVINGS

½ cup white wine vinegar
2 large cloves garlic, minced
1 piece (1 inch) fresh ginger, peeled and minced
1 tablespoon ground turmeric
2 teaspoons dry mustard
1½ teaspoons ground cumin
1 teaspoon ground coriander
½ teaspoon coarse salt
½ teaspoon freshly ground pepper
½ teaspoon (or less) cayenne pepper

½ teaspoon ground cardamom
½ teaspoon ground cinnamon
½ teaspoon ground cloves
1 shoulder or boneless leg of lamb (1½ pounds), cut into 1-inch cubes
1 tablespoon extra virgin olive oil
½ cup chopped yellow onion
1 cup chicken broth
½ cup coarsely chopped cilantro leaves

To make the Lamb Vindaloo Marinade, combine the white wine vinegar, garlic, ginger, turmeric, mustard, cumin, coriander, salt, pepper, cayenne, cardamom, cinnamon, and cloves in a large resealable plastic bag and blend well. Add the lamb and turn to coat all over. Seal the bag, and refrigerate for several hours or overnight, turning the lamb at least once.

(continues)

Heat a large skillet over medium heat for 2 minutes. Add the olive oil and swirl the pan to coat the bottom evenly. Add the onion and sauté for 4 minutes, stirring occasionally. Add the lamb and the Lamb Vindaloo Marinade and sauté over medium-high heat for 5 minutes, stirring frequently. Add the chicken broth and cilantro and bring to a boil. Cover, and simmer over low heat for 30 to 50 minutes or until the lamb is tender.

EACH SERVING PROVIDES:

6g carbohydrates, 301 calories, 36g protein, 14g fat,
2g dietary fiber, 584mg sodium, 109mg cholesterol

Pacific Rim Pork Tenderloin

If you like spicy foods infused with Asian ingredients, then this is the dish for you. The pork gets its heat from the chili paste, which is a combination of chilis, salt, and oil. I promise you, it will be worth the trip to the Asian food store to buy the chili paste. You will find yourself dreaming up ways to use it again and again. However, don't despair if you can't find it—simply substitute Sriracha hot chili sauce or a favorite hot pepper sauce. Serve with Asian Green Bean Stir-Fry (page 277).

4 SERVINGS

1 tablespoon soy sauce	1 teaspoon Asian sesame oil
1 tablespoon cold water	1 teaspoon chili paste
1 tablespoon rice vinegar	1 teaspoon hoisin sauce
1 tablespoon minced fresh ginger	1 clove garlic, minced
	1 pork tenderloin (1½ pounds)

To make the Pacific Rim Marinade, combine all ingredients except for the pork in a large resealable plastic bag and blend well. Add the pork tenderloin and turn to coat all over. Seal the bag, and refrigerate for several hours or overnight, turning the pork at least once.

Preheat oven to 325 degrees F. Lightly coat a shallow pan with a nonstick vegetable spray.

Remove the pork tenderloin from the marinade (reserve the marinade). Place the pork in the prepared pan. Bake for 45 to 55 minutes or until a meat thermometer registers 150 to 155 degrees F, basting the pork with the reserved marinade occasionally. Transfer the pork to a carving board and cover loosely with foil. Cool at least 10 minutes before carving it into thin slices.

To serve, place overlapping slices of pork on each of four dinner plates, dividing evenly among the servings.

(continues)

VEGETARIAN VARIATION: Substitute 1½ pounds extra firm tofu for the pork.

Place the tofu on a double thickness of paper towels and blot dry. Cut the tofu into four slices, each about ¾- to 1-inch thick. Place the tofu in a nonreactive dish and pour the marinade over the pieces. Turn to coat all over. Cover, and refrigerate for several hours.

Remove the tofu from the marinade (discard the marinade). Insert two wooden skewers (which have soaked in water for at least 30 minutes) parallel to each other into each piece of tofu. Cook the tofu on the grill for 5 to 8 minutes on each side or until golden brown. Or, place the tofu on a rimmed baking sheet that has been lightly coated with a nonstick vegetable spray. Preheat the oven to 375 degrees F and bake for 20 to 25 minutes.

EACH SERVING PROVIDES:
2g carbohydrates, 228 calories, 36g protein, 7g fat,
0g dietary fiber, 383mg sodium, 101mg cholesterol

Peppered Shrimp

If you like hot food then this signature dish was designed for you. The shrimp is cooked in a richly flavored butter sauce bursting with cayenne pepper. Of course, the amount of cayenne can be adjusted to suit your taste. This dish has an extra bonus in that the shrimp are cooked in their shells, leaving the peeling work to your hungry guests. Don't worry. For them it will be a labor of love.

4 SERVINGS

4 ounces (1 stick) butter
2 tablespoons fresh lemon juice
1 clove garlic, minced
1 teaspoon curry powder
½ teaspoon cayenne pepper
½ teaspoon dried oregano
   leaves

½ teaspoon coarse salt
½ teaspoon freshly ground
   pepper
1½ pounds large raw shrimp, in
   their shells

MELT the butter in a large skillet over low heat. Add the rest of the ingredients except the shrimp and blend well. Cook over medium-high heat for 5 to 10 minutes or until the sauce starts to brown, stirring constantly. Add the shrimp and turn to coat all over. Cook the shrimp for 5 to 7 minutes, stirring occasionally.

EACH SERVING PROVIDES:

2g carbohydrates, 378 calories, 36g protein, 25g fat,
0g dietary fiber, 620mg sodium, 394mg cholesterol

Sesame-Coated Salmon with Wasabi Sauce

This sesame-crusted salmon dish is a real taste treat. To further complement it, I like to make a sauce that includes wasabi to add some heat. Wasabi is a root that looks like horseradish but is smaller in size. This "hot" condiment is sold powdered in cans or as a paste in Asian food stores and in some supermarkets. If you use the powdered form, simply mix it with some water until it reaches a pastelike consistency.

4 SERVINGS

¼ cup nonfat cottage cheese
¼ cup whipping cream
2 tablespoons mayonnaise
1 tablespoon wasabi paste
1 tablespoon Dijon mustard
½ teaspoon Splenda or other artificial sweetener

¼ cup sesame seeds
4 salmon (or tuna) fillets (6 ounces each), skin removed
¼ cup extra virgin olive oil

To make the Wasabi Sauce, place the cottage cheese in the work bowl of a food processor fitted with a metal blade (or in a blender) and process until pureed. Add the whipping cream, mayonnaise, wasabi, mustard, and Splenda and blend well. Transfer the sauce to a covered dish and refrigerate until ready to serve.

Place the sesame seeds on a plate. Lightly brush the top of each salmon fillet with some of the olive oil. Dip the oiled side into the sesame seeds.

Heat a large nonstick skillet over medium-high heat for 1 minute. Add the remaining olive oil and swirl the pan to coat the bottom evenly. Add the salmon fillets, sesame seed side down, and cook for 5 minutes. Turn the salmon over and cook 5 minutes or until the salmon is no longer red when a knife is inserted into the thickest part.

To serve, spoon some Wasabi Sauce on each of four dinner plates. Place a salmon fillet in the center of the sauce.

EACH SERVING PROVIDES:

4g carbohydrates, 538 calories, 38g protein, 41g fat,
1g dietary fiber, 269mg sodium, 120mg cholesterol

Southwestern Shrimp with Creamy Chipotle Sauce

Chipotle chilies are dried jalapeños that have been smoked. They are intensely hot and have a characteristic smoky flavor. Pairing this "heated" sauce with shrimp that have been infused with the flavors of the Southwest doesn't get much better. Serve with Zesty Green Beans (page 310).

4 SERVINGS

½ cup nonfat cottage cheese
1 chipotle chili, minced*
1 recipe Southwestern
Marinade (page 214)

1½ pounds large raw shrimp,
peeled and deveined
4 sprigs fresh cilantro (optional)

To make the Creamy Chipotle Sauce, place the cottage cheese in the work bowl of a food processor fitted with a metal blade (or in a blender) and process until pureed. Add the chipotle chili and blend well. Transfer the sauce to a covered dish and refrigerate until 1 hour before serving.

Combine the Southwestern Marinade and shrimp in a large resealable plastic bag and turn to coat all over. Seal the bag, and refrigerate for 30 to 45 minutes, turning the shrimp at least once.

Meanwhile, soak wooden bamboo skewers (8 to 10 inches long) in enough water to cover.

When ready to grill, remove the shrimp from the marinade (discard the marinade). Thread the shrimp onto the skewers and place them on a grill coated with a nonstick vegetable spray over medium-hot coals. It is best to thread the shrimp on double-pronged skewers or two skewers that are parallel to each other, about 1 inch apart. This will pre-

---

*Chipotle chilis are very hot. You can control the heat of the sauce by adding more or less than the suggested amount.

vent the shrimp from spinning around when the skewer is turned, making it easier to cook them evenly on both sides. Cover the grill and cook for 3 minutes on each side.

To serve, remove the shrimp from the skewers and arrange them on each of four dinner plates. Spoon some Creamy Chipotle Sauce over each serving. Garnish with a sprig of cilantro, if desired.

Vegetarian Variation: Substitute 8 ounces tempeh, cut into 1½-inch cubes, for the shrimp.

EACH SERVING PROVIDES:

5g carbohydrates, 233 calories, 40g protein, 6g fat,
1g dietary fiber, 841mg sodium, 334mg cholesterol

ON THE GRILL

Who doesn't enjoy the intensely smoky flavor of foods that have been prepared on the grill? Grilling is not only for hamburgers and ribs but also for any food that can withstand the heat of the glowing coals while remaining tender and juicy. Best of all, imparting the smoky just-grilled flavor to your meat, poultry, seafood, or vegetables doesn't add unwanted calories or carbohydrates.

Butterflied Leg of Lamb

My favorite way to prepare a leg of lamb is to have it butterflied. Simply ask your butcher to remove the bone in the leg and to spread the meat so it will lie flat when cooked. Immersing it in a rosemary-infused marinade is a perfect combination of flavors.

6 SERVINGS

1 boneless leg of lamb
  (2¼ pounds), butterflied
3 tablespoons extra virgin
  olive oil
2 tablespoons garlic red wine
  vinegar
1½ tablespoons chopped fresh
  rosemary (or 1 tablespoon
  dried rosemary)

4 teaspoons fresh thyme leaves
  (or 2 teaspoons dried thyme
  leaves)
4 teaspoons fresh marjoram
  leaves (or 2 teaspoons dried
  marjoram leaves)
1 tablespoon cold water
½ teaspoon coarse salt
½ teaspoon freshly ground
  pepper

USING a meat mallet (or the bottom of a frying pan), pound the thicker portion of the lamb to the same thickness as the rest of the meat.

To make the Rosemary Marinade, combine the rest of the ingredients in a large resealable plastic bag and blend well. Add the lamb and turn to coat all over. Seal the bag, and refrigerate for several hours or overnight, turning the lamb at least once.

When ready to grill the lamb, remove it from the marinade (discard the marinade). Place the lamb on a grill coated with a nonstick vegetable spray over medium-hot coals. Sear the lamb for 1 minute on each side. Cover the grill and cook, turning the lamb every 10 minutes for 25 to 30 minutes or until a meat thermometer registers 150 degrees F for medium-rare or 160 degrees F for medium. Cool at least 10 minutes before carving it into thin slices.

(continues)

To serve, place overlapping slices of lamb on each of six dinner plates, dividing evenly among the servings.

VARIATION: To prepare the lamb in the oven: Preheat the oven to 350 degrees F, lightly coat a roasting pan with a nonstick vegetable spray, and place the lamb in the prepared pan. Bake for 35 to 45 minutes or until a meat thermometer registers 150 degrees F for medium-rare or 160 degrees F for medium.

EACH SERVING PROVIDES:

1g carbohydrates, 219 calories, 23g protein, 13g fat,
0g dietary fiber, 212mg sodium, 71mg cholesterol

ABOUT LAMB

Lamb comes from sheep that are less than two years old. A milk-fed lamb (sometimes called baby lamb) is between six and eight weeks old and was never weaned to eat grass or grain. This lamb will have an exceptionally sweet flavor and will be tender. A spring lamb is slightly older, between three and nine months, and has a mild flavor and tender meat. A yearling is between twelve and twenty-four months old, and its meat is tougher and gamier.

The most tender cuts of lamb come from the loin and rib section and include the lamb chop. There are two types of lamb chops. Rib lamb chops are the meatiest while shoulder and loin chops are less meaty and have more fat.

The plumpest legs of lamb have a higher ratio of meat to bone, making for a more tasty and tender cut of meat. The parchmentlike covering or "fell" on a leg of lamb helps retain its juices during grilling.

Cornish Hens with Jerk Rub

Cornish hens are so easy to prepare on the grill. All you need is a good pair of poultry shears for cutting down the backbone of the hen and then carefully opening it to lie flat to resemble a butterfly. The second most important necessity is a good rub, especially this one that adds an irresistible zip.

4 SERVINGS

1 tablespoon dried thyme leaves
1 tablespoon onion powder
2 teaspoons Splenda or other artificial sweetener
2 teaspoons ground allspice
2 teaspoons coarsely ground pepper

1 teaspoon coarse salt
½ teaspoon (or less) cayenne pepper
½ teaspoon ground nutmeg
¼ teaspoon ground cloves
2 Cornish hens (20 ounces each), butterflied

To make the Jerk Rub, combine all the ingredients except the hens in a small covered jar and blend well.

Place the Cornish hens in a large nonreactive dish. Spread the rub on both sides of the hens. Cover, and refrigerate for several hours or overnight.

To prepare the Cornish hens, place them on a grill coated with a nonstick vegetable spray over medium-hot coals. Cover the grill and cook, turning the hens frequently, for 20 to 25 minutes or until a meat thermometer placed in the thickest part of the thigh registers 180 degrees F.

To serve, cut each hen into two servings and place each one on a dinner plate.

(continues)

VARIATION: To prepare the Cornish hens in the oven: Preheat the oven to 450 degrees F, lightly coat a rimmed baking sheet with a non-stick vegetable spray, and place the hens on the prepared sheet. Bake for 15 minutes.

Reduce the oven temperature to 350 degrees F. Bake for 35 to 40 minutes or until a meat thermometer placed in the thickest part of the thigh registers 180 degrees F.

EACH SERVING PROVIDES:

4g carbohydrates, 442 calories, 49g protein, 25g fat,
1g dietary fiber, 1033mg sodium, 156mg cholesterol

Greek Chicken

This flavorful recipe for chicken is one of my favorites from my cookbook *The Complete Indoor/Outdoor Grill.* It is delicious when prepared on the grill but is equally savory when baked in an oven. All you need to complete this meal is a Greek Salad (page 142) and Greek Marinated Vegetable Kebabs (page 290).

4 SERVINGS

2 tablespoons Greek dried oregano leaves

1 tablespoon ground Greek oregano

2 teaspoons salt

2 teaspoons freshly ground pepper

1 teaspoon dried thyme leaves

1 large clove garlic, minced

1 whole chicken (3½ to 4 pounds), split along the backbone, and wing tips and all visible fat removed

To make the Greek Rub, combine all the ingredients except the chicken in a small bowl and blend well. Press the rub on both sides of the chicken. Place the chicken in an extra large resealable plastic bag (or a large nonreactive dish). Seal the bag, and refrigerate for several hours or overnight.

To prepare the chicken, place it on a grill coated with a nonstick vegetable spray over medium-hot coals. Cover the grill and cook, turning the chicken every 5 minutes, for 30 to 40 minutes or until a meat thermometer registers 180 degrees F. (The skin on the chicken may cause flare-ups. When you turn the chicken, make sure to extinguish any flames.)

To serve, cut the chicken into four servings and place each one on a dinner plate.

(continues)

VARIATION: To prepare the chicken in the oven: Preheat the oven to 375 degrees F, lightly coat a rimmed baking sheet with a nonstick vegetable spray, and place chicken on the baking sheet, breast side up. Bake for 20 minutes. Turn the chicken over and bake 15 minutes. Turn the chicken over to breast side up again and bake 40 minutes or until a meat thermometer inserted into the thickest part of the leg registers 180 degrees F.

EACH SERVING PROVIDES:

3g carbohydrates, 471 calories, 50g protein, 28g fat,

1g dietary fiber, 1092mg sodium, 156mg cholesterol

Grilled Mediterranean Lemon Chicken

The simplicity of this dish is a great example of how easy it is to prepare a delicious chicken breast by first marinating it in a lemony marinade and then grilling it to perfection. Pork, Cornish hens, or turkey fillets can be substituted for the chicken. Serve with a mixed green salad and Greek Marinated Vegetable Kebabs (page 290).

4 SERVINGS

¼ cup fresh lemon juice
1 large clove garlic, minced
1 tablespoon extra virgin olive oil
1½ teaspoons dried oregano leaves

½ teaspoon coarse salt
½ teaspoon freshly ground pepper
4 skinless and boneless chicken breast halves (6 ounces each)

To make the Lemon Marinade, combine all the ingredients except the chicken in a large resealable plastic bag and blend.

Place the chicken breasts between sheets of waxed paper. Pound them with a mallet (or the bottom of a frying pan) to flatten them to ½ inch. Place the chicken breasts in the marinade and turn to coat all over. Seal the bag, and refrigerate for several hours or overnight, turning the chicken at least once.

When ready to grill the chicken breasts, remove them from the marinade (discard the marinade). Place the chicken on a grill coated with a nonstick vegetable spray over medium-hot coals. Cover the grill and cook for 5 to 6 minutes on each side or until the juices run clear when the chicken is pierced with a fork.

(continues)

VARIATION: To broil the chicken breasts: Preheat the broiler, lightly coat a broiler pan with a nonstick vegetable spray, and place the chicken on the prepared pan. Broil, 4 to 5 inches from the heat source, for 5 to 6 minutes on each side or until the juices run clear when pierced with a fork.

EACH SERVING PROVIDES:

2g carbohydrates, 221 calories, 34g protein, 8g fat,
0g dietary fiber, 318mg sodium, 94mg cholesterol

Grilled Thai Shrimp with Dipping Sauce

Grilling shrimp marinated in a Thai-infused marinade accentuates the flavor of these tiny denizens of the sea. I like to serve them with Thai Dipping Sauce, but it is not an absolute. In fact, once you have tasted these tasty shrimp, you might consider using the marinade with chicken, Cornish hens, duck, or any other dish you can dream up. Serve with Green Beans with Cheese and Cashews (page 295).

4 SERVINGS

Thai Dipping Sauce
6 tablespoons rice vinegar
½ tablespoon Splenda
¼ teaspoon coarse salt
1 tablespoon finely chopped fresh cilantro leaves
1 tablespoon cold water
1 clove garlic, minced
¼ teaspoon dried red pepper flakes

Thai Marinade
3 tablespoons soy sauce
1 tablespoon canola oil
2 tablespoons fresh lemon juice
2 tablespoons chopped fresh cilantro leaves
1 clove garlic, minced
1 teaspoon minced fresh ginger
¼ teaspoon Sriracha hot chili sauce or favorite hot pepper sauce
1½ pounds large raw shrimp, peeled and deveined

To make the Thai Dipping Sauce, bring the rice vinegar, Splenda, and salt to a simmer in a small saucepan over medium heat, stirring occasionally. Simmer for 2 minutes. Remove the saucepan from the heat. Cool to room temperature.

Transfer the dipping sauce to a small bowl. Add the cilantro, water, garlic, and red pepper flakes and blend well. Cover, and set aside.

(continues)

To make the Thai Marinade, combine the ingredients in a large re-sealable plastic bag. Add the shrimp and turn to coat all over. Seal the bag, and refrigerate for 1 hour, turning the shrimp at least once.

When ready to grill the shrimp, remove them from the marinade (discard the marinade). Thread the shrimp onto 8- to 10-inch metal skewers (or wooden skewers that have soaked in water for at least 30 minutes). It is best to thread the shrimp on double-pronged skewers or two skewers that are parallel to each other, about 1 inch apart. This will prevent the shrimp from spinning around when the skewer is turned, making it easier to cook them evenly on both sides. Place the shrimp on a grill coated with a nonstick vegetable spray over medium-hot coals. Cover the grill and cook for 3 minutes on each side.

To serve, divide the Thai Dipping Sauce among four small bowls. Place the bowls on each of four dinner plates and arrange the shrimp kebabs beside them, dividing evenly among the servings.

EACH SERVING PROVIDES:

3g carbohydrates, 213 calories, 36g protein, 5g fat,
0g dietary fiber, 1295mg sodium, 332mg cholesterol

TO PEEL AND DEVEIN SHRIMP

When a recipe calls for peeled shrimp, start by removing the shell underneath where the legs are attached. To devein the shrimp, use a paring knife to make a shallow slit down the middle of the back to expose the black intestine. Remove the intestine by lifting it out with the point of the knife or simply rinsing it out under cold running water.

Lemon and Tarragon Marinated Salmon

This delightful salmon dish is so easy to prepare, yet it is simply delicious. The salmon derives its flavor from the aromatic Lemon and Tarragon Marinade, which also can be used to accent other seafood, such as tuna or swordfish. Be certain not to marinate the fish for more than 30 minutes because lemon juice can initiate a chemical change in fish similar to cooking. Serve with Mixed Baby Greens with Blue Cheese and Walnuts (page 143).

4 SERVINGS

¼ cup fresh lemon juice
1 tablespoon extra virgin
   olive oil
1 tablespoon fresh tarragon (or
   1 teaspoon dried tarragon
   leaves)
¼ teaspoon coarse salt

¼ teaspoon freshly ground
   pepper
4 salmon fillets (6 ounces each),
   skin removed
Thin slices of lemon, for
   garnish

To make the Lemon and Tarragon Marinade, combine all the ingredients except the salmon in a nonreactive dish and blend well. Add the salmon fillets and turn to coat all over. Cover, and refrigerate for 30 minutes, turning the salmon at least once.

When ready to grill the salmon fillets, remove them from the marinade (discard the marinade). Place the salmon on a grill coated with a nonstick vegetable spray over medium-hot coals. Cover the grill and cook for 10 minutes or until the salmon is no longer red when a knife is inserted into the thickest part.

To serve, place a salmon fillet on each of four dinner plates and garnish each with a slice of lemon, if desired.

(continues)

VARIATION: To broil the salmon fillets: Preheat the broiler, lightly coat a broiler pan with a nonstick vegetable spray, and place the salmon on the prepared pan. Broil the salmon, 4 to 5 inches from the heat source, for 5 to 6 minutes on each side or until the salmon is no longer red when a knife is inserted into the thickest part.

VEGETARIAN VARIATION: Substitute 1½ pounds extra firm tofu for the salmon.

Place the tofu on a double thickness of paper towels and blot dry. Cut the tofu into four slices, each about ¾- to 1-inch thick. Place the tofu in a nonreactive dish and pour the marinade over the pieces. Turn to coat all over. Cover, and refrigerate for several hours.

Remove the tofu from the marinade (discard the marinade). Insert two wooden skewers (that have soaked in water for at least 30 minutes) parallel to each other into each piece of tofu. Cook the tofu on the grill for 5 to 8 minutes on each side or until golden brown. (Or, pre-heat the oven to 375 degrees F, lightly coat a rimmed baking sheet with a nonstick vegetable spray, place the tofu on the prepared sheet, and bake for 20 to 25 minutes.)

EACH SERVING PROVIDES:
2g carbohydrates, 279 calories, 34g protein, 14g fat,
0g dietary fiber, 196mg sodium, 94mg cholesterol

Savory Rubbed Baby Back Ribs

In my home, nothing is more eagerly anticipated than these baby back ribs. My family absolutely adores them. I find that by keeping a container of rub readily available in the pantry, it makes preparing this low-carbohydrate family pleaser a snap. Serve with Cauliflower (sans Potato) Salad (page 141) and Zucchini Soufflé (page 316).

4 SERVINGS

1 tablespoon coarsely ground pepper

1 tablespoon paprika

1 tablespoon Splenda or other artificial sweetener

½ teaspoon celery salt

½ teaspoon dried oregano leaves

½ teaspoon coarse salt

½ teaspoon dried thyme leaves

½ teaspoon garlic salt

½ teaspoon (or less) cayenne pepper

2 slabs baby back pork ribs (3 pounds each)*

To make the Savory Rub, combine all the ingredients except the ribs in a small bowl and blend well.

Place the ribs in a large nonreactive pan. Prick the meat between the bones with a fork to tenderize them. Press a thick layer of rub on both sides of the ribs, if you like spicy foods, or apply a thin layer of the rub to make it less spicy. Cover, and refrigerate for several hours or overnight.

When ready to grill the ribs, place a grilling pan off to one side on the grilling grate and fill it with water. Place briquettes on the other half and light them. When the coals are medium hot, place the ribs on a grill coated with a nonstick vegetable spray over the grilling pan filled with

(continues)

*Ask your butcher to remove any thick layers of fat and to cut away both the membrane and the flap, or skirt, on the underside of the ribs.

water and away from the heat. (It is okay to stack the ribs. Alternate them after 1 hour of cooking time.) Cover the grill, leaving the vents on the lid slightly opened, and cook for 1½ to 2 hours or until a meat thermometer registers 150 to 155 degrees F. Check the temperature of the ribs after 1 hour and 15 minutes. The meat should easily pull apart when you pull the ribs in opposite directions or you should be able to insert a skewer between the bones easily.

EACH SERVING PROVIDES:

3g carbohydrates, 591 calories, 86g protein, 24g fat,
1g dietary fiber, 823mg sodium, 213mg cholesterol

Shish Kebab

I used to prepare shish kebabs by alternately threading chunks of lamb with a variety of vegetables. I have found, however, that it is better to grill the meat and vegetables separately because of the disparity in cooking time. Serve with Green Beans with Garlic and Red Pepper Flakes (page 296).

6 SERVINGS

¼ cup fresh lemon juice
¼ cup chopped yellow onion
1 large clove garlic, chopped
2 tablespoons extra virgin
    olive oil
2 teaspoons dry mustard
½ teaspoon coarse salt
½ teaspoon freshly ground
    pepper
1 shoulder or boneless leg of
    lamb (2¼ pounds), cut into
    1½-inch cubes

1 yellow onion, cut into 6 to 12
    wedges
1 green bell pepper, cut into
    1-inch squares
1 red bell pepper, cut into
    1-inch squares
6 to 12 large fresh button
    mushrooms

To make the Shish Kebab Marinade, combine the lemon juice, onion, garlic, olive oil, mustard, salt, and pepper in a large resealable plastic bag and blend well. Add the lamb and turn to coat all over. Seal the bag, and refrigerate for several hours or overnight, turning the lamb at least once.

When ready to grill the lamb, remove it from the marinade (discard the marinade). Thread the lamb cubes onto metal skewers (or wooden skewers that have soaked in water for at least 30 minutes) and the vegetables onto separate skewers. Or, alternately thread lamb, onion, peppers, and mushrooms onto the skewers. It is best to thread the lamb

(continues)

and vegetables on double-pronged skewers or two skewers that are parallel to each other, about 1 inch apart. This will prevent the lamb and vegetables from spinning around when the skewer is turned, making it easier to cook them evenly on both sides. Place the skewers on a grill coated with a nonstick vegetable spray over medium-hot coals. Cover the grill and cook for 8 to 12 minutes or until a meat thermometer registers 150 degrees F for medium-rare or 160 degrees F for medium, turning the skewers at least once.

EACH SERVING PROVIDES:

7g carbohydrates, 311 calories, 36g protein, 15g fat,
2g dietary fiber, 243mg sodium, 109mg cholesterol

Southwestern Rubbed Flank Steak

Coating flank steak with this spicy rub before cooking adds an authentic Southwestern flavor. The steak is especially delicious topped with traditional fajita fixings, such as sauéed onions, green peppers, sour cream, cheese, or salsa.

4 SERVINGS

1 tablespoon ground cumin
½ tablespoon chili powder
½ tablespoon Splenda or other artificial sweetener
2 teaspoons ground coriander
1 teaspoon dry mustard
1 teaspoon coarsely ground pepper

1 teaspoon dried oregano leaves
½ teaspoon coarse salt
¼ teaspoon (or more) cayenne pepper
1 flank steak (1½ pounds), pierced all over with a fork

To make the Southwestern Rub, combine all the ingredients except the steak in a small bowl and blend well.

Place the flank steak in a nonreactive dish. Spread the rub on both sides of the flank steak. Cover, and refrigerate for several hours or overnight.

To prepare the flank steak, place it on a grill coated with a nonstick vegetable spray over medium-hot coals. Sear the steak for 1 minute on each side. Cover the grill and cook for 5 to 6 minutes on each side or until a meat thermometer registers 145 degrees F. Carve the flank steak across the grain into very thin diagonal slices.

VARIATION: To broil the flank steak: Preheat the broiler, lightly coat a broiler pan with a nonstick vegetable spray, and place the steak on the prepared pan. Broil, 4 to 5 inches from the heat source, for 4 to 5 minutes on each side or until a meat thermometer registers 145 degrees F.

EACH SERVING PROVIDES:
2g carbohydrates, 288 calories, 36g protein, 14g fat,
1g dietary fiber, 357mg sodium, 88mg cholesterol

Swordfish with Olive and Red Pepper Relish

Swordfish benefits from being marinated before cooking it on the grill. To further add interest, I like to top it with a Greek-accented red pepper and olive relish. This colorful condiment would also nicely highlight the flavor of other seafood, such as tuna and salmon. Serve with a Greek Salad (page 142).

6 SERVINGS

1 red bell pepper
1 cup chopped Greek olives
   (Kalamatas)
1 tablespoon minced fresh
   parsley
1 tablespoon capers, rinsed and
   drained
1 tablespoon extra virgin
   olive oil

1 clove garlic, minced
1 teaspoon red wine vinegar
½ recipe Greek Vinaigrette
   (page 142)
3 swordfish steaks (12 ounces
   each)

To make the Olive and Red Pepper Relish, place the red pepper on a baking sheet lined with aluminum foil. Broil the pepper under a preheated broiler, turning the pepper as the skin blackens, for 20 to 25 minutes or until the skin is charred all over. Once the pepper is roasted, place it in a resealable plastic bag, seal, and allow it to steam for 15 to 20 minutes. When the pepper is cool enough to handle, peel away the skin and remove the top and seeds. (Do not rinse the pepper.) Dice the pepper.

Combine the diced red pepper, olives, parsley, capers, olive oil, garlic, and red wine vinegar in a bowl and blend well. Cover, and refrigerate for several hours or overnight. Stir before serving.

Place the Greek Vinaigrette in a large nonreactive dish and add the swordfish steaks. Turn to coat both sides. Cover, and refrigerate for 30 minutes, turning the swordfish at least once.

When ready to grill the swordfish steaks, remove them from the marinade (discard the marinade). Place the swordfish on a grill coated with a nonstick vegetable spray over medium-hot coals. Cover the grill and cook for 10 minutes or until the swordfish is no longer translucent when a knife is inserted into the thickest part.

To serve, divide each swordfish steak into two servings and place each one on a dinner plate. Spoon some of the Olive and Red Pepper Relish on top or to the side of each serving.

EACH SERVING PROVIDES:

5g carbohydrates, 425 calories, 35g protein, 29g fat,
1g dietary fiber, 891mg sodium, 66mg cholesterol

Tandoori Chicken

In India, many people prepare game hens in a tandoor, which is a pitlike red clay oven that can reach intense temperatures, as high as 900 degrees F. I have found that my Weber grill is almost as good at creating this succulent dish.

4 SERVINGS

1 cup plain yogurt
2 tablespoons fresh lime juice
1 piece (2 inches) fresh ginger, peeled and minced
1 large clove garlic, minced
1 teaspoon chili powder
1 teaspoon coarse salt
¼ teaspoon ground cumin

¼ teaspoon ground turmeric
1 tablespoon tandoori paste or a few drops red food coloring (optional)
1 whole chicken (3½ to 4 pounds), split along the backbone, and wing tips and all visible fat removed

To make the Tandoori Chicken Marinade, combine all the ingredients except the chicken in an extra large resealable plastic bag (or a large nonreactive dish) and blend well. Add the chicken and turn to coat all over. Seal the bag, and refrigerate for several hours or overnight, turning the chicken at least once.

When ready to grill the chicken, remove it from the marinade (reserve the marinade). Place the chicken on a grill coated with a nonstick vegetable spray over medium-hot coals. Cover the grill and cook for 30 to 40 minutes or until a meat thermometer registers 180 degrees F, turning the chicken every 5 minutes and basting one or two times with the marinade. (The skin on the chicken may cause flare-ups. When you turn the chicken, make sure to extinguish the flames.)

VARIATION: To prepare the chicken in the oven: Preheat the oven to 375 degrees F, lightly coat a rimmed baking sheet with a nonstick vegetable spray, place the chicken on the baking sheet, breast side up, and bake for 20 minutes. Turn the chicken over and bake another 20 minutes. Turn the chicken again and bake 25 minutes or until a meat thermometer inserted into the thickest part of the leg registers 180 degrees F.

EACH SERVING PROVIDES:
4g carbohydrates, 503 calories, 52g protein, 30g fat,
0g dietary fiber, 656mg sodium, 164mg cholesterol

Tex-Mex Flank Steak
with Gazpacho Salsa

This flavorful flank steak, adorned with Gazpacho Salsa, is in the highest tradition of the Southwest. When I know I am going to make a Beef Fajita Salad (page 114), I usually double the amount of flank steak and marinade. By doubling the recipe, I can use the leftovers to create this special main course.

4 SERVINGS

1 flank steak (1½ pounds), pierced all over with a fork

Southwestern Marinade
¼ cup fresh lime juice
1 tablespoon extra virgin olive oil
1 large clove garlic, minced
1 teaspoon ground cumin
1 teaspoon dried oregano leaves
¾ teaspoon coarse salt
½ teaspoon chili powder
⅛ teaspoon cayenne pepper

Gazpacho Salsa
¼ cup diced red bell pepper
¼ cup diced yellow bell pepper
¼ cup diced red onion
¼ cup diced and seeded tomato
1 tablespoon chopped fresh cilantro leaves
1 clove garlic, minced
1 jalapeño pepper, seeded and minced*
½ tablespoon extra virgin olive oil
1 teaspoon sherry vinegar

To make the Southwestern Marinade, combine all the ingredients in a large resealable plastic bag and blend. Add the flank steak and turn to coat all over. Seal the bag, and refrigerate for several hours or overnight, turning the steak at least once.

*The seeds of a jalapeño pepper are very hot. To avoid burning your skin, wear rubber or latex gloves when removing the seeds. Immediately wash the knife, cutting surface, and gloves when finished.

To make the Gazpacho Salsa, combine all the ingredients in a small dish and blend well. Cover, and refrigerate for up to 6 hours.

When ready to grill the flank steak, remove it from the marinade (discard the marinade). Place the steak on a grill coated with a non-stick vegetable spray over medium-hot coals. Sear the steak for 1 minute on each side. Cover the grill and cook for 5 to 6 minutes on each side or until a meat thermometer registers 145 degrees F. Carve the flank steak across the grain into very thin diagonal slices.

VARIATION: To broil the flank steak: Preheat the broiler, lightly coat a broiler pan with a nonstick vegetable spray, and place the steak on the prepared pan. Broil, 4 to 5 inches from the heat source, for 4 to 5 minutes on each side or until a meat thermometer registers 145 degrees F.

EACH SERVING PROVIDES:
6g carbohydrates, 343 calories, 36g protein, 19g fat,
1g dietary fiber, 460mg sodium, 88mg cholesterol

Tuna Fajitas

Grilled tuna reaches a new dimension by marinating it with the flavors of the Southwest. When topped with a fabulous Tomatillo Salsa and traditional fajita fixin's, you'll never miss the tortilla. All you need to complete the meal is a salad accented with a Southwestern Vinaigrette (page 114).

4 SERVINGS

Tomatillo Salsa
3 tomatillos
½ tablespoon extra virgin
  olive oil
½ cup packed chopped fresh
  cilantro leaves
2 jalapeño peppers, seeded*
1 clove garlic, minced
3 tablespoons fresh lime juice
¼ teaspoon coarse salt
½ cup plain yogurt

Lime Juice Marinade
¼ cup fresh lime juice
¼ cup packed finely chopped
  fresh cilantro leaves
½ tablespoon extra virgin
  olive oil

1 clove garlic, chopped
⅛ teaspoon coarse salt
⅛ teaspoon freshly ground
  pepper

4 tuna steaks (6 ounces each)
1½ tablespoons extra virgin
  olive oil
½ cup thinly sliced yellow onion
1 medium green bell pepper,
  thinly sliced
2 diced and seeded Roma
  tomatoes, for garnish

*The seeds of a jalapeño pepper are very hot. To avoid burning your skin, wear rubber or latex gloves when removing the seeds. Immediately wash the knife, cutting surface, and gloves when finished.

To make the Tomatillo Salsa, peel off the husks and stems of the tomatillos. Wash them under hot running water to remove the sticky resinous material covering the tomatillos. Thinly slice the tomatillos.

Heat a small frying pan over medium heat for 2 minutes. Add ½ tablespoon olive oil and swirl the pan to coat the bottom evenly. Add the tomatillos and sauté for 4 minutes, stirring frequently. Set aside.

In the work bowl of a food processor fitted with a metal blade (or in a blender), process ½ cup cilantro, jalapeños, and garlic until finely chopped. Add the tomatillos and blend well. Add 3 tablespoons lime juice, ¼ teaspoon coarse salt, and yogurt and pulse just until blended. Transfer the Tomatillo Salsa to a covered container and refrigerate for up to 4 hours. Taste for seasoning before serving.

To make the Lime Juice Marinade, combine the ¼ cup lime juice, ¼ cup cilantro, ½ tablespoon olive oil, garlic, and ⅛ teaspoon salt and pepper in a nonreactive dish. Add the tuna steaks and turn to coat both sides. Cover, and refrigerate for 30 minutes.

Meanwhile, pour ½ tablespoon olive oil into a plastic bag. Add the onion and green pepper slices and turn to coat all over.

Place a large nonstick skillet over medium heat for 2 minutes. Add the vegetables and sauté for 7 to 8 minutes or until soft, stirring occasionally. Remove the skillet from the heat. Cover, and set aside.

When ready to grill the tuna steaks, remove them from the marinade (discard the marinade). Place the tuna on a grill coated with a nonstick vegetable spray over medium-hot coals. Cover the grill and cook for 5 minutes on each side or until the tuna is no longer red when a knife is inserted into the thickest part.

To serve, place a tuna steak on each of four dinner plates. Spoon some Tomatillo Salsa over each serving and top with the sautéed onions and green peppers, dividing evenly among the servings. Garnish each serving with tomatoes.

(continues)

VARIATION: To sauté the tuna steaks, heat a large nonstick skillet over medium-high heat for 1 minute. Add 1 tablespoon olive oil and swirl the pan to coat the bottom evenly. Add the tuna steaks and cook for 4 to 5 minutes on each side or until no longer opaque when a knife is inserted into the thickest part.

EACH SERVING PROVIDES:

11g carbohydrates, 454 calories, 53g protein, 21g fat,
2g dietary fiber, 289mg sodium, 87mg cholesterol

ABOUT TOMATILLOS

Tomatillos are Mexican green tomatoes that resemble cherry tomatoes but are firmer, juicier, and more tart. They will turn yellow if allowed to ripen; the preferred way to use them is when they are green. Tomatillos are found in the produce section of most supermarkets.

EXOTIC FLAVORS

Take a gourmet trip around the world by sampling some of the exotic international flavors included in this section. Start your culinary odyssey in Thailand and consider gastronomic side trips to Morocco and India. Each of these recipes is your passport to an exciting adventure in low-carbohydrate dining.

Asian Rubbed Salmon

This rub not only enriches the flavor of salmon but it can also be used to adorn pork, poultry, or beef. If you have a favorite Asian-inspired sauce, spoon some over the salmon once it is cooked. Serve with Asian Green Bean Stir-Fry (page 277).

4 SERVINGS

½ tablespoon ground coriander
½ tablespoon coarsely ground pepper
½ tablespoon Chinese Five Spice powder
½ tablespoon Splenda or other artificial sweetener

½ teaspoon coarse salt
⅛ teaspoon dried red pepper flakes
4 salmon fillets (6 ounces each), skin removed

To make the Asian Rub, combine all the ingredients except the salmon in a small jar and blend well. (The rub can be made ahead and stored in a covered container until ready to use.)

To prepare the salmon fillets, preheat the broiler, lightly coat a broiler pan with a nonstick vegetable spray, place the salmon on the prepared pan, and spread the rub on both sides. Broil, 4 to 5 inches from the heat source, for 4 to 5 minutes on each side or until the salmon is no longer red when a knife is inserted into the thickest part.

VARIATION: To grill the salmon fillets, place them on a grill coated with a nonstick vegetable spray over medium-hot coals. Cover the grill and cook for 10 minutes or until the salmon is no longer red when a knife is inserted into the thickest part.

EACH SERVING PROVIDES:
2g carbohydrates, 248 calories, 34g protein, 11g fat,
0g dietary fiber, 311mg sodium, 94mg cholesterol

ABOUT SALMON

Salmon is a firm, pink-fleshed fish with a delicate, butter-smooth flavor and texture. It is sold as either Atlantic salmon or Pacific salmon, the former being the tastier, especially if caught in Scotland or Ireland. Pacific salmon usually are harvested wild, so they are available only during the spring and summer months.

Caribbean Rubbed Flank Steak

Once you have tasted flank steak coated with this spicy Caribbean Rub, you won't be able to wait for an excuse to try it on pork, chicken, or anything else. You also will be glad you tried the Pickapeppa sauce, a Jamaican condiment made from mangoes, cane vinegar, raisins, peppers, and tamarind and found in the steak sauce section of most supermarkets.

6 SERVINGS

½ tablespoon ground allspice
½ tablespoon coarse salt
½ tablespoon coarsely ground pepper
½ tablespoon ground nutmeg
½ tablespoon ground cinnamon
½ tablespoon ground ginger
½ tablespoon Splenda or other artificial sweetener

1 teaspoon dried thyme leaves
½ teaspoon onion powder
½ teaspoon garlic powder
⅛ teaspoon ground cloves
1 tablespoon Pickapeppa sauce
1 tablespoon (or more) cold water
1 flank steak (2¼ pounds), pierced all over with a fork

To make the Caribbean Rub, combine the allspice, salt, pepper, nutmeg, cinnamon, ginger, Splenda, thyme, onion powder, garlic powder, and cloves in a small bowl. Add the Pickapeppa sauce and enough water to make a paste and blend well.

Place the flank steak in a nonreactive dish. Spread the rub on both sides of the steak. Cover, and refrigerate for several hours or overnight.

Preheat the broiler, lightly coat a broiler pan with a nonstick vegetable spray, and place the flank steak on the prepared pan. Broil, 4 to 5 inches from the heat source, for 4 to 5 minutes on each side or until a meat thermometer registers 145 degrees F. Carve the flank steak across the grain into very thin slices.

To serve, place overlapping slices of steak on each of six dinner plates, dividing evenly among the servings.

VARIATION: To grill the flank steak, place it on a grill coated with a nonstick vegetable spray over medium-hot coals. Sear the steak for 1 minute on each side. Cover the grill and cook for 5 to 6 minutes on each side or until no longer red when a knife is inserted into the thickest part.

EACH SERVING PROVIDES:

3g carbohydrates, 285 calories, 36g protein, 14g fat,

1g dietary fiber, 601mg sodium, 88mg cholesterol

Cornish Hens with Thai Rub

Coating Cornish hens with this Asian-inspired rub results in a fusion of delectable flavors. Once you have tasted this spectacular dish, you might want to experiment by using the rub on ribs, pork, or even salmon. Serve with Sesame Broccoli (page 304).

4 SERVINGS

½ tablespoon Splenda or other artificial sweetener

2 teaspoons dried lemon peel

2 teaspoons ground coriander

1½ teaspoons onion salt

1 teaspoon garlic salt

1 teaspoon ground ginger

1 teaspoon freshly ground pepper

1 teaspoon ground cumin

1 teaspoon (or less) cayenne pepper

2 Cornish hens (20 ounces each), butterflied

To make the Thai Rub, combine all the ingredients except the Cornish hens in a small covered jar and blend well.

Place the Cornish hens in a large nonreactive dish. Spread the rub on both sides of the hens. Cover, and refrigerate for several hours or overnight.

Preheat oven to 450 degrees F. Lightly coat a rimmed baking sheet with a nonstick vegetable spray. Place the Cornish hens on the baking sheet and bake for 15 minutes.

Reduce oven temperature to 350 degrees F. Bake for 45 to 50 minutes or until a meat thermometer registers 180 degrees F.

To serve, cut each hen into two servings and place each one on a dinner plate.

VARIATION: To grill the Cornish hens, place them on a grill coated with a nonstick vegetable spray over medium-hot coals. Cover the grill and cook, turning the hens frequently, for 20 to 25 minutes or until a meat thermometer placed in the thickest part of the thigh registers 180 degrees F.

EACH SERVING PROVIDES:

2g carbohydrates, 435 calories, 49g protein, 24g fat,

1g dietary fiber, 1694mg sodium, 156mg cholesterol

ABOUT CORNISH HENS

Cornish hens are small broiler chickens that are produced by crossing a Cornish, bantam, or small cock with a white Plymouth rock hen. Cornish hens also are called Cornish rock hens, rock Cornish hens, or Cornish game hens. At five to six weeks of age, they weigh from one to two pounds.

Cuban Pork Loin Roast

One of my favorite ways to prepare a pork roast is to marinate it in a tart mixture that includes many of the ingredients typically found in Cuban cuisine. This marinade also tenderizes the meat, resulting in a richly flavorful and succulent low-carbohydrate delight. Serve with Zucchini and Green Olive Medley (page 313).

8 SERVINGS

⅓ cup fresh orange juice
2 tablespoons fresh lime juice
1 tablespoon extra virgin olive oil
1 large clove garlic, minced
1 teaspoon ground cumin

1 teaspoon dried oregano leaves
1 teaspoon coarse salt
½ teaspoon freshly ground pepper
1 pork loin boneless roast (3 pounds), trimmed and tied

To make the Orange Juice Marinade, combine all the ingredients except the pork in a large resealable plastic bag and blend well.

Add the pork roast and turn to coat all over. Seal the bag, and refrigerate for several hours or overnight, turning the pork at least once.

Preheat oven to 325 degrees F. Place the pork roast in a roasting pan and pour the marinade over the top. Bake, basting with the pan juices occasionally, for 2 hours or until a meat thermometer inserted into the center of the pork registers 145 to 150 degrees F. (Add additional orange juice to the roasting pan if it becomes dry.) Transfer the pork to a carving board and cover loosely with foil. Cool at least 10 minutes before carving it into thin slices.

To serve, place overlapping slices of pork on each of eight dinner plates, dividing evenly among the servings.

EACH SERVING PROVIDES:

3g carbohydrates, 369 calories, 52g protein, 15g fat,
0g dietary fiber, 459mg sodium, 133mg cholesterol

Lemongrass Marinated Whole Chicken

Including lemongrass in the marinade imparts a subtle, lemony flavor to this Asian-inspired chicken dish. The marinade also can be used to enhance the flavor of Cornish hens, as well as cut-up chickens. Serve with Sesame Broccoli (page 304).

4 SERVINGS

1 whole chicken (3½ to 4 pounds), wing tips removed
3 minced lemongrass stalks, ends trimmed and outer covering removed
3 tablespoons canola oil
2 tablespoons cold water

1 clove garlic, minced
1 tablespoon soy sauce
1 teaspoon Splenda or other artificial sweetener
1 teaspoon (or more) dried red pepper flakes
1 teaspoon coarse salt

USING poultry shears, cut down the backbone of the chicken and then carefully open it to lie flat, resembling a butterfly. Remove all visible fat and organs. Rinse well and pat dry with paper towels.

To make the Lemongrass Marinade, combine the rest of the ingredients in a large resealable plastic bag (or a large nonreactive dish) and blend well. Add the chicken and turn to coat all over. Seal the bag, and refrigerate for several hours or overnight, turning the chicken at least once.

Preheat oven to 375 degrees F. Lightly coat a rimmed baking sheet with a nonstick vegetable spray.

Remove the chicken from the marinade (reserve the marinade). Place the chicken on the prepared pan, breast side up, and bake for 20 minutes. Turn the chicken over and bake 15 minutes. Turn the chicken

(continues)

over to breast side up again and bake, basting at least once with the marinade, for another 40 minutes or until a meat thermometer inserted into the thickest part of the leg registers 180 degrees F.

To serve, cut the chicken into four servings and place each one on a dinner plate.

VARIATION: To grill the chicken, place it on a grill coated with a nonstick vegetable spray over medium-hot coals. Cover the grill and cook, turning the chicken every 5 minutes, for 30 to 40 minutes or until a meat thermometer inserted into the thickest part of the leg registers 180 degrees F. (The skin on the chicken may cause flare-ups. When you turn the chicken, make sure to extinguish the flames.)

EACH SERVING PROVIDES:

2g carbohydrates, 555 calories, 50g protein, 38g fat,
0g dietary fiber, 851mg sodium, 156mg cholesterol

ABOUT LEMONGRASS

Lemongrass is a Southeast Asian herb. Its fibrous outer layer is removed to reveal the inner stalk, which is the culinary heart of the plant. It has a delicate lemon flavor that seems to embrace food with a subtle citrus perfume. Look for fresh lemongrass in the produce section of many supermarkets.

Mediterranean Turkey Patties

Combining ground turkey with a mélange of Mediterranean spices results in a highly flavorful taste sensation. It is delicious when topped with a spoonful of Greek Yogurt and Cucumber Dip (Tsatziki) (page 57) and served with a Greek Salad (page 142) alongside. I like to make extra patties to enjoy as a satisfying low-carbohydrate lunch the next day.

6 SERVINGS

2¼ pounds ground turkey
½ cup finely minced yellow
  onion
3 tablespoons minced fresh
  cilantro leaves
1 large clove garlic, minced
4 teaspoons ground cumin
2 teaspoons ground coriander
1 teaspoon coarse salt

1 teaspoon freshly ground
  pepper
½ teaspoon cayenne pepper
¼ teaspoon ground allspice
¼ teaspoon ground cinnamon
¼ teaspoon ground ginger
2 tablespoons extra virgin
  olive oil

USING clean hands, combine all the ingredients except the olive oil in a large bowl until well blended. (The turkey mixture can be refrigerated in a covered container for several hours or overnight.)

Form the turkey mixture into 6 patties.

Heat a large skillet over medium-high heat for 1 minute. Add the olive oil and swirl the pan to coat the bottom evenly. Add the turkey patties and sauté for 4 to 5 minutes on each side or until cooked through.

To serve, place a turkey patty on each of six dinner plates and top with a dollop of Greek Yogurt and Cucumber Dip (Tsatziki), if desired.

(continues)

VARIATION: To grill the turkey patties, place them on a grill coated with a nonstick vegetable spray over medium-hot coals. Cover the grill and cook for 4 to 5 minutes on each side.

EACH SERVING PROVIDES:

3g carbohydrates, 329 calories, 32g protein, 22g fat,

1g dietary fiber, 535mg sodium, 146mg cholesterol

Moroccan Chicken with Sliced Almonds

Preparing chicken in this Moroccan-inspired sauce allows it to absorb the wonderfully exotic complement of spices seldom enjoyed west of Casablanca. For ease of preparation, you can simmer the chicken a day ahead and allow it to sit in the sauce overnight. This step also allows the complexity of flavors to intensify.

4 SERVINGS

1 tablespoon extra virgin olive oil
½ cup chopped yellow onion
1 cup cold water (or chicken broth)
½ teaspoon ground cinnamon
½ teaspoon ground ginger
½ teaspoon ground cumin
½ teaspoon ground turmeric
½ teaspoon ground coriander

½ ¾ teaspoon freshly ground pepper
½ teaspoon coarse salt
¼ teaspoon saffron threads (or 1½ teaspoon saffron powder)
2 tablespoons fresh lemon juice
1 cut-up chicken (3½ pounds) *or 4 thighs*
6 tablespoons sliced almonds
~~4 sprigs fresh cilantro~~

HEAT a Dutch oven or large skillet over low heat for 2 minutes. Add the olive oil and swirl the pan to coat the bottom evenly. Add the onion. Cover, and cook for 5 minutes. Add the water *broth*, cinnamon, ginger, cumin, turmeric, coriander, pepper, salt, saffron, and lemon juice and blend well. Add the chicken. Bring to a boil. Cover, and simmer over medium-low heat for 30 minutes, turning the chicken over after 15 minutes. (At this point, you can refrigerate the dish for completion later. Cover the Dutch oven and refrigerate for up to 24 hours.)

(continues)

Preheat oven to 350 degrees F. Lightly coat a rimmed baking sheet with a nonstick vegetable spray. Place the chicken (reserve the sauce, and taste for seasoning) on the baking sheet. Pour enough sauce over the chicken to coat the pieces evenly. Distribute the almonds over the top. Bake for 30 minutes.

Meanwhile, reheat the reserved sauce in a small saucepan over medium-low heat, stirring occasionally. Taste for seasoning.

To serve, place a chicken breast on each of four dinner plates and spoon some sauce over each serving. Garnish with cilantro, if desired.

EACH SERVING PROVIDES:

5g carbohydrates, 984 calories, 98g protein, 61g fat,
2g dietary fiber, 528mg sodium, 302mg cholesterol

New Delhi Turkey Meatloaf

This is a very special meatloaf. It is infused with many of the spices frequently found in Indian cuisine. On the subject of spices, feel free to add heaping spoonfuls of them for a spicier flavor. I like to serve this hearty dish with Green Beans with Cheese and Cashews (page 295).

6 SERVINGS

2 tablespoons extra virgin
   olive oil
½ cup chopped yellow onion
1 clove garlic, minced
1 teaspoon curry powder
½ teaspoon ground ginger
½ teaspoon coarse salt
½ teaspoon freshly ground
   pepper

½ teaspoon ground coriander
¼ teaspoon ground cumin
¼ teaspoon ground cinnamon
¼ teaspoon cayenne pepper
1½ pounds ground turkey
1 egg, lightly beaten
1 teaspoon Dijon mustard

PREHEAT oven to 325 degrees. Lightly coat a 9 × 5-inch loaf pan with a nonstick vegetable spray. Set aside.

Heat a medium nonstick skillet over medium heat for 2 minutes. Add the olive oil and swirl the pan to coat the bottom evenly. Add the onion, garlic, curry, ginger, salt, pepper, coriander, cumin, cinnamon, and cayenne and sauté for 5 minutes, stirring occasionally. Remove the skillet from the heat. Cool at least 10 minutes.

Using your hands, combine the turkey, onion mixture, egg, and mustard in a large bowl and blend well. Place the turkey mixture in the prepared pan and press down on the top to make it evenly flat. Bake

(continues)

for 80 to 90 minutes. Remove the turkey meatloaf from the oven and carefully drain off as much fat as possible. Serve immediately by cutting the meatloaf into slices and placing a serving on each of six dinner plates.

EACH SERVING PROVIDES:

2g carbohydrates, 247 calories, 22g protein, 17g fat,
1g dietary fiber, 334mg sodium, 133mg cholesterol

Pacific Rim Marinated Salmon

If you have shied away from eating fresh seafood, you will be cured of this aversion quickly after one taste of this delectable salmon. This incredible marinade can be used to enhance the flavors of most seafood as well as meat, poultry, and tofu. I like to serve the salmon on a bed of Zucchini Pasta (page 315).

4 SERVINGS

¼ cup soy sauce
2 tablespoons chopped green onion
1 tablespoon Splenda or other artificial sweetener
1 tablespoon minced fresh ginger
1 tablespoon minced garlic
4 salmon fillets (6 ounces each), skin removed
12 strands of fresh chives for garnish (optional)

LIGHTLY coat a broiler pan with a nonstick vegetable spray. Set aside.

To make the Teriyaki Marinade, combine all the ingredients except the salmon in a nonreactive dish and blend well. Add the salmon fillets and turn to coat all over. Cover, and refrigerate for 1 hour, turning the salmon at least once.

Preheat the broiler. Remove the salmon fillets from the marinade (discard the marinade) and place them on the prepared pan. Broil, 4 to 5 inches from the heat source, for 4 to 5 minutes on each side or until the salmon is no longer red inside when a knife is inserted into the thickest part.

To serve, place a salmon fillet on each of four dinner plates. Garnish each serving with long strands of chives, if desired.

(continues)

VARIATION: To grill the salmon fillets, place them on a grill coated with a nonstick vegetable spray over medium-hot coals. Cover the grill and cook for 10 minutes or until the salmon is no longer red inside when a knife is inserted into the thickest part.

EACH SERVING PROVIDES:

4g carbohydrates, 262 calories, 35g protein, 11g fat,
0g dietary fiber, 1105mg sodium, 94mg cholesterol

Veal Piccata

This subtle lemon-flavored Italian dish is surprising for its simplicity and is destined to become a favorite. As veal can be very costly, I frequently substitute chicken breasts flattened to ½ inch in thickness. Serve with Broccoli with Garlic and Cheese (page 283).

4 SERVINGS

2 tablespoons extra virgin
olive oil
4 veal scallops (6 ounces each)
½ teaspoon coarse salt
½ teaspoon freshly ground
pepper
1 large clove garlic, minced
½ cup chicken broth
¼ cup fresh lemon juice

2 tablespoons capers, rinsed and
drained
2 tablespoons butter, at room
temperature
2 tablespoons minced fresh
parsley
4 thin slices of lemon, for
garnish

HEAT a large skillet over medium-high heat for 1 minute. Add the olive oil and swirl the pan to coat the bottom evenly. Season both sides of the veal with salt and pepper. Place the veal in a single layer in the skillet and sauté for 2 to 2½ minutes on each side or until lightly browned. (It may be necessary to sauté half the veal at a time.) Remove the veal to a plate and cover loosely with aluminum foil.

Add the garlic to the skillet and sauté for about 30 seconds or until fragrant. Add the chicken broth and cook over high heat for 2 minutes, scraping the bottom of the skillet with a wooden spoon to loosen any browned bits. Add the lemon juice and capers and cook for 1 minute. Remove the skillet from the heat and add the butter. Swirl the pan until the butter melts. Add the parsley and blend.

(continues)

To serve, place a veal scallop on each of four dinner plates. Spoon some sauce over the veal, dividing evenly among the servings. Garnish each serving with a lemon slice, if desired.

EACH SERVING PROVIDES:

2g carbohydrates, 325 calories, 32g protein, 20g fat,
1g dietary fiber, 595mg sodium, 141mg cholesterol

IN THE MAIN

If you were a meat-and-potatoes devotee, take heart! Even though you will have to cross potatoes off your menu list, you will find that the centerpiece meat, poultry, and seafood entrées featured here, infused with wonderful spices, herbs, and marinades, will stand alone and satisfy without the embellishment of starchy vegetables.

Beef Tenderloin with Mushroom Sauce

When you want to impress your friends, serve this elegant beef tenderloin smothered in a creamy mushroom sauce. Who would believe such a masterful entrée could be so delicious and low in carbohydrates at the same time. Serve with Sesame Broccoli (page 304).

4 SERVINGS

3 tablespoons soy sauce

2 tablespoons rice wine

1 teaspoon Dijon mustard

⅛ teaspoon freshly ground pepper

1 beef tenderloin (1½ pounds)

1 tablespoon butter, at room temperature

1 cup whipping cream

1 tablespoon Asian sesame oil

2 tablespoons canola oil

1 tablespoon minced fresh ginger

8 ounces sliced fresh button or shiitake mushrooms

12 strands of fresh chives, for garnish

PREHEAT oven to 400 degrees F. Lightly coat a shallow pan with a nonstick vegetable spray.

Combine 1 tablespoon soy sauce, 1 tablespoon rice wine, mustard, and pepper in a small bowl and blend well. Set aside.

Place the beef tenderloin in the prepared pan. Spread the butter over the top of the beef. Bake for 20 minutes.

After 20 minutes, brush the beef with the soy sauce mixture. Bake for an additional 25 to 30 minutes or until a meat thermometer registers 145 degrees F, basting occasionally. Remove the beef tenderloin from the oven. Cover loosely with aluminum foil.

To make the Mushroom Sauce, combine the whipping cream, the remaining 2 tablespoons soy sauce, the remaining 1 tablespoon rice wine, and sesame oil in a small bowl and blend well.

Heat a medium skillet over medium heat for 2 minutes. Add the canola oil and ginger and swirl the pan to coat the bottom evenly. Add the mushrooms and sauté for 2 to 3 minutes or until tender. Add the whipping cream mixture and bring to a boil over medium-high heat. Boil for 3 to 6 minutes or until the sauce thickens, stirring occasionally.

To serve, carve the beef tenderloin into slices and place them on each of four dinner plates, dividing evenly among the servings. Spoon some Mushroom Sauce over each serving. Garnish with long strands of chives, if desired.

EACH SERVING PROVIDES:

6g carbohydrates, 622 calories, 39g protein, 48g fat,
1g dietary fiber, 908mg sodium, 195mg cholesterol

ABOUT BEEF

When buying beef, look for brightly colored, red to deep red cuts with a moderate amount of marbling. Leaner cuts of meat tend to be less tender and less tasty. However, marinating them for several hours or overnight in a liquid or paste mixture will tenderize them as well as add flavor. A useful rule of thumb to follow when looking for leaner cuts of beef is to look for the words loin or round in the name. The leanest cuts are the beef eye round, top round, round tip, top sirloin, and tenderloin.

Test for doneness by inserting a meat thermometer to measure the temperature of the thickest part of the meat or by observing the color of the beef through a slit made near its center. If the thermometer registers 120 to 135 degrees F or if the center is bluish-maroon and the outer portion is pale brown, then the meat is rare. If the thermometer registers 135 to 140 degrees F or if the center is deep red and the outer portion is light to medium brown, then it is medium rare. A temperature of 140 to 150 degrees F or a light pink center and medium to dark brown outer portion, indicates that it is medium. A reading of 155 to 165 degrees F or beef that appears uniformly brown throughout suggests that the meat is well done.

Cornish Hens with Lemon Glaze

If you love the flavor of lemon, you will adore a Cornish hen glazed with this heavenly tart sauce. The sauce can be made a day ahead, and preparing the chicken is effortless. Serve with Brussels Sprouts with Cardamom (page 284).

4 SERVINGS

½ cup fresh lemon juice
2 tablespoons extra virgin
  olive oil
½ teaspoon white wine vinegar
1 clove garlic, minced
⅛ teaspoon dried oregano
  leaves

⅛ teaspoon coarse salt
⅛ teaspoon freshly ground
  pepper
2 Cornish hens (20 ounces
  each), butterflied

To make the Lemon Sauce, combine all the ingredients except the hens in a medium bowl and blend well. Cover, and refrigerate for several hours or overnight. (Stir the sauce before using.)

Preheat the broiler, lightly coat a broiler pan with a nonstick vegetable spray, and place the Cornish hens on the pan. Broil, 6 inches from the heat source and turning the hens every 10 minutes, for 35 to 40 minutes or until a meat thermometer placed in the thickest part of the thigh registers 180 degrees F.

Remove the Cornish hens from the broiler and brush both sides with the Lemon Sauce. Return the hens to the broiler for 3 minutes on each side.

To serve, cut each hen into two servings and place each one on a dinner plate.

EACH SERVING PROVIDES:

3g carbohydrates, 497 calories, 49g protein, 31g fat,
0g dietary fiber, 619mg sodium, 156mg cholesterol

Curried Mustard-Coated Flank Steak

Get ready for rave reviews from family and friends when you serve this flavorful steak. Not only is it delicious but the steak also can be marinated the evening before, which makes it quick and easy. Serve with Cauliflower Puree (page 287).

4 SERVINGS

2 tablespoons butter, at room temperature
2 tablespoons Dijon mustard
1 teaspoon curry powder
1 teaspoon Worcestershire sauce
½ teaspoon coarse salt

½ teaspoon freshly ground pepper
1 flank steak (1½ pounds), pierced all over with a fork
¼ cup Madeira wine

COMBINE the butter, mustard, curry, Worcestershire sauce, salt, and pepper in a small bowl and blend well or until it is the consistency of mayonnaise.

Place the flank steak in a nonreactive dish. Spread the butter mixture on the top of the flank steak and pour the Madeira over it. Cover, and refrigerate for several hours or overnight.

Preheat the broiler, lightly coat a broiler pan with a nonstick vegetable spray, and place the flank steak on the pan. Broil, 4 to 5 inches from the heat source, for 4 to 5 minutes on each side or until a meat thermometer registers 145 degrees F. Carve the flank steak across the grain into very thin diagonal slices.

To serve, place overlapping slices of steak on each of four dinner plates, dividing evenly among the servings.

(continues)

VARIATION: To grill the flank steak, place it on a grill coated with a nonstick vegetable spray over medium-hot coals. Sear the steak for 1 minute on each side. Cover the grill and cook for 5 to 6 minutes on each side or until a meat thermometer registers 145 degrees F.

EACH SERVING PROVIDES:

3g carbohydrates, 439 calories, 47g protein, 24g fat,
0g dietary fiber, 580mg sodium, 130mg cholesterol

Lemon Chicken

This is one of my favorite ways to serve chicken. The lemon juice marries so well with the seasoned chicken, and, best of all, it only takes minutes to produce this ambrosial delight.

6 SERVINGS

6 skinless and boneless chicken breast halves (6 ounces each)

¾ teaspoon freshly ground pepper

½ teaspoon coarse salt

6 tablespoons butter

2 tablespoons extra virgin olive oil

¼ cup finely chopped fresh parsley

2 tablespoons fresh lemon juice

6 lemon slices, for garnish (optional)

Sprigs of parsley, for garnish (optional)

PREHEAT the oven to 250 degrees F. Place the chicken breasts between sheets of waxed paper. Pound them with a mallet (or the bottom of a frying pan) to flatten them to ½ inch. Sprinkle both sides of the chicken breasts with pepper and salt.

Melt 2 tablespoons butter in a large skillet over moderate heat. Add the olive oil and blend. Increase the heat to medium high and add the chicken breasts. Sauté for 5 to 6 minutes on each side or until the juices run clear when pierced with a fork.

Place the chicken breasts in a baking dish. Cover loosely with foil and keep warm in the oven while you prepare the lemon sauce.

To make the Lemon Sauce, melt 4 tablespoons butter in the same skillet over medium heat, scraping up any brown bits with a wooden spoon. Remove the skillet from the heat and add the parsley and lemon juice. Blend well.

(continues)

To serve, place the chicken breasts on each of six dinner plates and spoon some Lemon Sauce over each serving, dividing evenly among the servings. Garnish each serving with a lemon slice and a sprig of parsley, if desired.

EACH SERVING PROVIDES:

1g carbohydrates, 439 calories, 37g protein, 31g fat,
0g dietary fiber, 248mg sodium, 149mg cholesterol

Maytag Blue Cheese Stuffed Pork Chops

Stuffing a pork chop with a delectable Maytag Blue Cheese filling is the closest thing to being in "hog heaven." If you double the amount of mushroom and green onions called for in the recipe, you can set aside half of the cooked mixture to spoon over the finished pork chop. Serve with Asparagus with Mustard Sauce (page 279).

6 SERVINGS

2 tablespoons extra virgin olive oil

½ cup thinly sliced fresh button mushrooms

¼ cup finely minced yellow onion

6 ounces Maytag Blue Cheese or favorite blue cheese, crumbled

¼ teaspoon coarse salt

⅛ teaspoon freshly ground pepper

6 thick-cut (1 to 1½ inches) pork loin chops

PREHEAT oven to 325 degrees F. Heat a medium skillet over medium heat for 2 minutes. Add the olive oil and swirl the pan to coat the bottom evenly. Add the mushrooms and onion and sauté for 4 minutes, stirring frequently. Remove the skillet from the heat and add the cheese, salt, and pepper and blend well. Set aside.

Cut a deep pocket in each pork chop by making a small incision at the small end of the chop and carefully rotating the blade inside the chop, keeping the opening no wider than 1 inch. Stuff the blue cheese mixture in the pork chop, dividing evenly. Place the pork chops in a shallow pan and bake for 45 minutes.

To serve, place a pork chop on each of six dinner plates and top with a dollop of the Maytag Blue Cheese filling, if desired.

EACH SERVING PROVIDES:

2g carbohydrates, 238 calories, 24g protein, 14g fat,

0g dietary fiber, 512mg sodium, 73mg cholesterol

Mustard-Coated Leg of Lamb

Serving tender slices of lamb coated with a flavorful mustard top-ping is an elegant meal to share during family gatherings or the holidays. It marries well with almost any of your favorite low-carbohydrate vegetables and salads. Simply start the meal by serving steaming bowls of Mushroom and Green Onion Soup (page 95) and sit back and wait for the rave reviews.

6 SERVINGS

¼ cup Dijon mustard
1 tablespoon soy sauce
½ tablespoon extra virgin
    olive oil
½ teaspoon dried thyme leaves

¼ teaspoon ground ginger
¼ teaspoon coarse salt
1 boneless leg of lamb (2¼
    pounds)

PREHEAT oven to 450 degrees F. Combine all the ingredients except the lamb in a small bowl and blend well.

Place the lamb in a roasting pan. Spread the mustard mixture over the top and sides of the lamb. (At this point, the lamb can be covered loosely with aluminum foil and refrigerated for several hours.)

Bake for 15 minutes. Reduce oven temperature to 350 degrees F. Bake for 1 hour and 30 minutes or until a meat thermometer registers 150 degrees F for medium-rare or 160 degrees F for medium. (Add about ½ to 1 cup water to the pan after 1 hour of baking time.) Cool at least 10 minutes before carving it into thin slices.

To serve, place overlapping slices of lamb on each of six dinner plates, dividing evenly among the servings.

EACH SERVING PROVIDES:
2g carbohydrates, 177 calories, 23g protein, 8g fat,
0g dietary fiber, 557mg sodium, 71mg cholesterol

Original Joe's Special

Original Joe's is a restaurant located in San Jose, California. Established in 1956, it is renowned for its large portions and honest Italian cooking. I have been serving an adaptation of this special dish to my family for years, and they still love it.

4 SERVINGS

1 pound prewashed spinach
2 tablespoons extra virgin
   olive oil
½ cup chopped yellow onion
1 pound lean ground beef
¾ teaspoon coarse salt
½ teaspoon dried basil

½ teaspoon freshly ground
   pepper
¼ teaspoon dried marjoram
   leaves
¼ teaspoon dried oregano
   leaves
4 eggs, lightly beaten

BRING 1 cup water to a boil in a large skillet over high heat. Add the spinach. Cover, and cook over low heat for 4 minutes. Transfer the spinach to a colander and drain well. When the spinach is cool enough to handle, place it in a towel and squeeze out as much moisture as possible. Chop the spinach and set aside. (The spinach can be prepared a day ahead. Place it in a covered container and refrigerate.)

Heat a large skillet over medium heat for 2 minutes. Add the olive oil and swirl the pan to coat the bottom evenly. Add the onion and sauté for 5 minutes, stirring occasionally. Add the beef and sauté for 5 to 10 minutes or until no longer pink, stirring frequently. Add the salt, basil, pepper, marjoram, oregano, and spinach and blend well. Cook until heated through, stirring frequently. Add the eggs and cook, without stirring, for 30 to 60 seconds or until the eggs are set. Taste for seasoning. Serve immediately.

EACH SERVING PROVIDES:

7g carbohydrates, 363 calories, 33g protein, 23g fat,
4g dietary fiber, 588mg sodium, 254mg cholesterol

Poached Salmon with Mustard Dill Sauce

Poaching is one of the easiest ways to prepare a salmon. When topped with a creamy dill sauce, this simple dish becomes a culinary treat. Serve with Green Beans with Hazelnuts (page 297).

4 SERVINGS

2 tablespoons Dijon mustard

1½ tablespoons white wine vinegar

½ teaspoon Splenda or other artificial sweetener

2 tablespoons minced fresh dill (or 2¼ teaspoons dried dill weed)

2 tablespoons extra virgin olive oil

1½ tablespoons whipping cream

½ teaspoon fresh lemon juice (optional)

¼ teaspoon coarse salt

¼ teaspoon freshly ground pepper

4 salmon fillets (6 ounces each), skin removed

Sprigs of dill, for garnish (optional)

To make the Mustard Dill Sauce, combine the mustard, vinegar, and Splenda in a jar with a tight-fitting lid and blend. Add the rest of the ingredients except the salmon. Cover the jar and shake to blend well. (The Mustard Dill Sauce can be made a day ahead. Cover and refrigerate. Bring to room temperature before using.)

Place the salmon fillets in a microwave-proof dish and add ¼ cup cold water. Cover the dish with a piece of plastic wrap and cook on high for 8 to 10 minutes or until the salmon is no longer red when a knife is inserted into the thickest part.

To serve, place a salmon fillet on each of four dinner plates. Spoon some Mustard Dill Sauce over each serving, dividing evenly among the servings. Garnish with a sprig of dill, if desired.

EACH SERVING PROVIDES:

1g carbohydrates, 334 calories, 34g protein, 21g fat,

0g dietary fiber, 385mg sodium, 101mg cholesterol

Pork Chops with Red Peppers

Quickly sautéing seasoned pork chops is a treat by itself, but for added color and taste, I like to top them with these savory red pepper strips. These red marvels are also delicious served on top of grilled lamb, swordfish, a hearty steak, or any other culinary creation you can imagine.

4 SERVINGS

4 tablespoons extra virgin olive oil
2 large red bell peppers, cut into thin strips
1 large clove garlic, minced
2 teaspoons fresh rosemary (or 1 teaspoon dried rosemary)
10 fresh sage leaves, chopped (or 1 teaspoon dried sage leaves)
¼ teaspoon coarse salt

¼ teaspoon freshly ground pepper
¼ cup white wine
4 loin pork chops (6 ounces each)
½ teaspoon coarse salt
½ teaspoon freshly ground pepper
Sprigs of dill for garnish (optional)

HEAT a large nonstick skillet over medium heat for 2 minutes. Add 2 tablespoons olive oil and swirl the pan to coat the bottom evenly. Add the red peppers. Cover, and cook for 5 minutes. Add the garlic, rosemary, sage, ¼ teaspoon salt, and ¼ teaspoon pepper and cook for 30 seconds, stirring constantly. Add the wine and bring to a boil over high heat. Remove the skillet from the heat. Cover loosely with aluminum foil and set aside.

Season both sides of the pork chops with the remaining salt and pepper. Heat a large nonstick skillet over medium heat for 2 minutes. Add 2 tablespoons olive oil and swirl the pan to coat the bottom evenly. Add the pork chops and sauté for 5 minutes on each side.

(continues)

Masterful Main Courses
••••

To serve, place a pork chop on each of four dinner plates. Spoon some red peppers over each serving, dividing evenly among the servings. Add sprigs of dill for garnish, if desired.

EACH SERVING PROVIDES:

6g carbohydrates, 316 calories, 25g protein, 20g fat,

2g dietary fiber, 429mg sodium, 70mg cholesterol

Salmon Glazed with Dill Butter

A friend gave me this recipe for a delicious way to prepare salmon. It can be served chilled but is equally delicious fresh from the oven. The salmon also could be used to create a main course salad by simply adding greens, a savory vinaigrette, and any of your favorite low-carbohydrate salad fixin's.

4 SERVINGS

3 tablespoons butter, melted
3 tablespoons chopped fresh
   dill
½ teaspoon coarse salt

¼ teaspoon freshly ground
   pepper
4 salmon fillets (6 ounces each),
   skin removed

PREHEAT oven to 500 degrees F. Line a rimmed baking sheet with a piece of parchment paper or lightly coat with a nonstick vegetable spray.

Combine the butter and dill in a small dish.

Season the salmon fillets with salt and pepper. Brush the tops of each with the butter mixture. Bake for 10 to 14 minutes or until the salmon is no longer red when a knife is inserted into the thickest part or when a meat thermometer registers 140 degrees F. (Cooking time will vary according to the thickness of the salmon.)

To serve, place a salmon fillet on each of four dinner plates. Garnish each serving with a sprig of dill, if desired.

EACH SERVING PROVIDES:
0g carbohydrates, 318 calories, 34g protein, 19g fat,
0g dietary fiber, 312mg sodium, 117mg cholesterol

Salmon with Saffron Vinaigrette

Sautéing salmon fillets creates an instant culinary treat, and fusing it with a Saffron Vinaigrette elevates this impressive seafood dish to an even higher taste sensation. Serve with Zucchini and Swiss Cheese Soufflé (page 317).

4 SERVINGS

3 tablespoons fresh lemon juice
1 tablespoon Dijon mustard
1 teaspoon Splenda or other
    artificial sweetener
⅛ teaspoon saffron threads (or
    1 teaspoon saffron powder)
½ cup extra virgin olive oil
4 salmon fillets (6 ounces each),
    skin removed

½ teaspoon coarse salt
½ teaspoon freshly ground
    pepper
2 tablespoons extra virgin
    olive oil
Fresh chives, for garnish

To make the Saffron Vinaigrette, place the lemon juice, mustard, Splenda, and saffron in the work bowl of a food processor fitted with a metal blade (or in a blender) and process until blended.

Add ½ cup olive oil in a slow, steady stream and process until smooth. (The Saffron Vinaigrette can be made a day ahead. Store in a covered container in the refrigerator. Stir before using and taste for seasoning.)

Season both sides of the salmon fillets with the salt and pepper.

Heat a large nonstick skillet over medium-high heat for 1 minute. Add 2 tablespoons olive oil and swirl the pan to coat the bottom evenly. Add the salmon fillets and sauté for 4 to 5 minutes on each side or until no longer red inside when a knife is inserted into the thickest part.

To serve, drizzle Saffron Vinaigrette on each of four dinner plates, dividing evenly among the servings. Place a salmon fillet in the center of the vinaigrette. Garnish each serving with long strands of chives, if desired.

EACH SERVING PROVIDES:

2g carbohydrates, 565 calories, 34g protein, 46g fat,
0g dietary fiber, 405mg sodium, 94mg cholesterol

ABOUT SAFFRON

Saffron is reputed to be the most expensive spice in the world. It is the dried stigma (the female part of the flower, found in the center) of the blue flower *Crocus sativus*. This flower is grown in Spain, India, and Turkey. Each flower produces three very small, deep-yellow-orange stigma threads that can be removed only by hand. It takes between 70,000 and 225,000 flowers to produce 1 pound of saffron.

This valued spice adds a golden color as well as a subtle but exotic aroma and flavor to dishes. Fortunately, a little saffron goes a long way.

Spicy Chicken Thighs

Spicy Chicken Thighs are absolutely delicious. For the ultimate taste sensation, spoon some Pine Nut Dip (page 68) over each serving and garnish with a sprig of cilantro. Serve with Zucchini and Green Olive Medley (page 313).

4 SERVINGS

4 tablespoons extra virgin
  olive oil
½ teaspoon chili powder
½ teaspoon ground cumin
½ teaspoon paprika

½ teaspoon coarse salt
½ teaspoon freshly ground
  pepper
12 to 16 chicken thighs

To make the Spicy Marinade, combine 2 tablespoons olive oil, chili powder, cumin, paprika, salt, and pepper in a large resealable plastic bag. Add the chicken thighs and turn to coat all over. Seal the bag, and refrigerate the chicken for several hours or overnight.

Preheat oven to 425 degrees F. Heat a large nonstick skillet over medium heat for 2 minutes. Add the remaining olive oil and swirl the pan to coat the bottom evenly. Add the chicken thighs and sauté for 3 minutes on each side. (It may be necessary to sauté half the chicken at a time.) Remove the chicken thighs to a baking dish. Bake for 30 minutes or until a meat thermometer registers 178 degrees F.

To serve, place equal servings of chicken thighs on each of four dinner plates.

EACH SERVING PROVIDES:
1g carbohydrates, 444 calories, 41g protein, 30g fat,
0g dietary fiber, 353mg sodium, 149mg cholesterol

Spicy Lamb Chops

Although my family is perfectly content to be served unadorned lamb chops, every now and then I like to add some spices to complement the dominant flavor of lamb. Although I broil the lamb chops in this recipe, they would be equally delectable if cooked on the grill.

4 SERVINGS

2 teaspoons ground cumin
1 teaspoon coarse salt
1 teaspoon ground cinnamon

½ teaspoon freshly ground
   pepper
1½ pounds lamb chops (loin
   or rib)

COMBINE the cumin, salt, cinnamon, and pepper on a plate and blend well.

Rub the spices on both sides of the lamb chops. (If not preparing the lamb chops immediately, cover and refrigerate for several hours or overnight.)

Preheat the broiler, lightly coat a broiler pan with a nonstick vegetable spray, and place the lamb chops on the pan. Broil, 4 to 5 inches inches from the heat source, for 7 to 8 minutes on each side or until a meat thermometer registers 150 degrees F for medium-rare or 160 degrees F for medium. Serve immediately by dividing lamb chops evenly and placing them on four dinner plates.

VARIATION: To grill the lamb chops, place them on a grill that has been coated with a nonstick vegetable spray over medium-hot coals. Cover the grill and cook for 4 to 5 minutes on each side.

EACH SERVING PROVIDES:
1g carbohydrates, 168 calories, 23g protein, 8g fat,
0g dietary fiber, 536mg sodium, 71mg cholesterol

STRICTLY VEGETARIAN

Vegetarian and low-carbohydrate dieting are not natural companions because so many vegetables have a high-carbohydrate content. However, with a little imagination, a touch of garlic, or an infusion of the right spices, low-carbohydrate vegetable staples such as zucchini, spinach, tofu, or tempeh can be transformed into amazingly delicious offerings.

Curried Tempeh with Spinach

Combining the nutty flavor of tempeh with a richly flavored curry sauce is the ultimate vegetarian meal. Although tempeh tends to be somewhat higher in carbohydrates than other soybean products, its fiber-rich and nutrient-filled qualities readily compensate for this. Serve with Zucchini Pasta (page 315).

4 TO 6 SERVINGS

6 cups prewashed baby spinach
1 can (14 ounces) pure "lite" coconut milk
1 package (8 ounces) tempeh, cut into ½-inch cubes
½ cup chopped yellow onion
3 red (or green) jalapeño peppers, seeded and minced*

2 bay leaves
1 large clove garlic, minced
1 teaspoon curry powder
1 teaspoon Splenda or other artificial sweetener
Chopped peanuts (optional)

COMBINE all the ingredients except the peanuts in a large skillet and blend. Bring to a boil over medium high heat. Cover, and simmer over low heat for 15 minutes. Remove the bay leaves. To serve, divide the curried tempeh among the dinner plates and garnish each serving with chopped peanuts, if desired.

EACH SERVING PROVIDES:
18g carbohydrates, 193 calories, 14g protein, 10g fat,
5g dietary fiber, 65mg sodium, 0mg cholesterol

(continues)

*The seeds of a jalapeño pepper are very hot. To avoid burning your skin, wear rubber or latex gloves when removing the seeds. Immediately wash the knife, cutting surface, and gloves when finished.

ABOUT TEMPEH

• •

Tempeh (pronounced TEMpay) is an Indonesian food. This soybean cake is produced by inoculating cooked soybeans with a mushroomlike culture and then placing it in a warm, dark place for a specified amount of time. Once the tempeh is ready, it is refrigerated. Tempeh has a chewy consistency and a nutty flavor. It can be steamed, grilled, used in stir-fry, or added to sauces. In fact, tempeh can be used pound for pound in place of ground meat. Look for tempeh in the freezer section of health food stores or in the health section of most supermarkets. Once tempeh is defrosted, you can store it in the refrigerator for up to 10 days.

Indonesian Tempeh

Tempeh is a traditional Indonesian food. These chunky cakes of soybeans can be crumbled and then cooked with a variety of flavorful ingredients to create a fiber-rich, tasty delight.

2 TO 3 SERVINGS

1 tablespoon canola oil
½ cup chopped yellow onion
1 tablespoon minced fresh
   ginger
1 clove garlic, minced
1 jalapeño pepper, minced*
¼ teaspoon ground turmeric
1 package (8 ounces) tempeh,
   crumbled or diced

1½ tablespoons soy sauce
¼ teaspoon (or more) dried red
   pepper flakes
¼ cup chopped peanuts
1 diced and seeded Roma
   tomato (optional)

HEAT a large skillet over medium heat for 2 minutes. Add the canola oil and swirl the pan to coat the bottom evenly. Add the onion, ginger, garlic, jalapeño, and turmeric and sauté for 5 minutes, stirring occasionally. Add the tempeh, soy sauce, and red pepper flakes and blend well. Cook for 2 minutes, stirring occasionally. Add the peanuts and optional tomato and blend. Cook for 1 minute.

EACH SERVING PROVIDES:
29g carbohydrates, 413 calories, 27g protein, 24g fat,
8g dietary fiber, 781mg sodium, 0mg cholesterol

*The seeds of a jalapeño pepper are very hot. To avoid burning your skin, wear rubber or latex gloves when removing the seeds. Immediately wash the knife, cutting surface, and gloves when finished.

Orange-Scented Tofu Stir-Fry

Combining tofu with a mélange of vegetables and an orange sauce creates a fabulous vegetarian dish that is not only nutritious but absolutely delicious! Feel free to substitute any of your favorite low-carbohydrate vegetables for the ones that I have suggested.

4 SERVINGS

1 box (12 ounces) extra firm tofu

¼ cup fresh orange juice

2 tablespoons soy sauce

1 tablespoon rice vinegar

½ teaspoon Splenda or other artificial sweetener

1 teaspoon Asian sesame oil

¼ teaspoon coarse salt

¼ teaspoon Sriracha or favorite hot pepper sauce

2 tablespoons canola oil

½ bunch bok choy, thinly sliced

1 cup broccoli florets

3 ounces fresh shiitake (or button) mushrooms, stemmed and thinly sliced

1 red bell pepper, thinly sliced

PLACE the tofu on a double thickness of paper towels and blot dry. Cut into ½-inch cubes. Set aside.

To make the Orange Stir-Fry Sauce, combine the orange juice, soy sauce, rice vinegar, Splenda, sesame oil, salt, and Sriracha in a small bowl and blend well. Set aside.

Heat a wok or large skillet over medium-high heat for 1 minute. Add the canola oil and swirl the pan to coat the bottom evenly. Add the bok choy, broccoli, mushrooms, and red pepper and stir-fry for 5 minutes or until the vegetables are crisp-tender. Add the Orange Stir-Fry Sauce and blend well. Allow the sauce to boil for 2 minutes. Add the tofu, and stir-fry until heated through.

EACH SERVING PROVIDES:

11g carbohydrates, 165 calories, 10g protein, 10g fat,

3g dietary fiber, 766mg sodium, 0mg cholesterol

Portobello Eggplant Pizzas

These giant mushrooms are mature cremini mushrooms. Not only are they intensely flavorful, these versatile behemoths can be baked, braised, grilled, and roasted, and they are simply delicious when made into a satisfying pizza. Although Portobello mushrooms can be topped with an infinite number of low-carbohydrate ingredients, I have chosen a recipe that is my favorite.

2 SERVINGS

4 Portobello mushrooms (5 to 6 inches in diameter), stems removed

4 tablespoons extra virgin olive oil

1 eggplant (8 ounces), cut into ¼- to ½-inch-thick rounds

¼ cup freshly grated Parmesan cheese

1 to 2 Roma tomatoes, cut into 8 to 12 thin rounds

¾ teaspoon fresh thyme (or ¼ teaspoon dried thyme leaves)

¼ teaspoon coarse salt

¼ teaspoon freshly ground pepper

PREHEAT oven to 375 degrees F. Coat a rimmed baking sheet with a nonstick vegetable spray. Use a damp paper towel to clean the Portobello mushrooms.

Heat a large skillet over medium heat for 2 minutes. Add 2 tablespoons olive oil and swirl the pan to coat the bottom evenly. Add the Portobello mushrooms and cook on both sides for 5 minutes. Transfer the mushrooms to a double thickness of paper towels and set aside.

Meanwhile, brush the eggplant rounds with the remaining olive oil. Place them on the prepared baking sheet and bake for 20 minutes or until tender. Turn the slices over and bake 5 minutes. Transfer the eggplant to a plate.

(continues)

To make the eggplant pizzas, place the Portobello mushrooms on the baking sheet. Sprinkle each mushroom with Parmesan cheese, dividing evenly. Arrange the tomato slices, slightly overlapping each other, on the mushrooms and top with overlapping slices of eggplant. Season each with thyme, salt, and pepper. Bake for 10 minutes.

VARIATION: To make roasted red pepper pizzas, follow the instructions for cooking the Portobello mushrooms. Top each cooked mushroom with half of a roasted red pepper found in Spicy Roasted Red Pepper Soup (page 101). Place two large fresh basil leaves on each red pepper and then sprinkle 6 to 8 tablespoons grated mozzarella cheese over each pizza, dividing evenly. Bake the pizzas as above or until the cheese has melted.

EACH SERVING PROVIDES:
20g carbohydrates, 402 calories, 14g protein, 32g fat,
11g dietary fiber, 501mg sodium, 10mg cholesterol

Roasted Vegetable Torte with Harissa Vinaigrette

Roasting vegetables is the ultimate way to intensify their flavors and inherently rich sweetness. Once cooked, the vegetables are simply layered in a dish to form a torte. This delectable torte is finished off with a drizzle of Harissa Vinaigrette over the top. Harissa is a Moroccan hot chili paste that is available in most Asian food stores or other food specialty shops. Serve with a Greek Salad (page 142).

4 TO 6 SERVINGS

*Harissa Vinaigrette**
½ cup extra virgin olive oil
2 tablespoons red wine vinegar
1 teaspoon Dijon mustard
1 teaspoon harissa sauce
½ teaspoon coarse salt
⅛ teaspoon freshly ground
   pepper

Roasted Vegetable Torte
2 large red bell peppers, halved
   and seeded
¼ to ½ cup extra virgin olive oil

½ teaspoon coarse salt
½ teaspoon freshly ground
   pepper
1 eggplant (1¼ pounds), cut
   into ½-inch-thick rounds
2 large Portobello mushrooms,
   stemmed and cleaned with a
   damp paper towel
3 zucchini (8 ounces each), cut
   lengthwise into ½-inch-thick
   slabs
4 ounces feta or goat cheese
   (optional)

To make the Harissa Vinaigrette, combine all the ingredients in a small jar with a tight-fitting lid. Shake well to blend. Set aside.

Preheat oven to 400 degrees F. Line two rimmed baking sheets with aluminum foil and heavily coat them with olive oil.

(continues)

*A zesty vinaigrette can be substituted for the Harissa Vinaigrette.

To make the Roasted Vegetable Torte, place the red peppers on a prepared baking sheet and brush both sides with some of the olive oil. Season with some of the salt and pepper. Roast for 20 minutes on each side or until tender. Transfer the peppers to a plate. Cut each pepper in half and cover loosely with aluminum foil. Set aside.

Place the eggplant, Portobello mushrooms, and zucchini on the baking sheets and brush both sides with the remaining olive oil. Season with salt and pepper. Bake for 15 to 20 minutes or until tender. (Cooking time will vary for individual vegetables. Periodically check the vegetables and remove those that are done to the plate containing the red peppers.)

To make the torte, use a sharp knife to thinly slice the Portobello mushrooms on the diagonal, as you would a brisket or flank steak.

Place the eggplant slices, slightly overlapping each other, on the bottom of an 8- or 9-inch pie plate that has been lightly coated with a non-stick vegetable spray. Alternate the zucchini and mushroom slices, in spokelike fashion, on top of the eggplant and then top with the red peppers. Cover the torte with a piece of waxed paper and place a pie pan on top. Gently press down on the top pie pan to flatten the torte. Remove the top pie pan and waxed paper. Cover the dish with plastic wrap and refrigerate for several hours or overnight.

To serve, cut the torte into wedges and place each one on a dinner plate. Place a piece of cheese off to the side, if desired. Drizzle Harissa vinaigrette over each serving.

EACH SERVING PROVIDES:
23g carbohydrates, 480 calories, 6g protein, 43g fat,
9g dietary fiber, 521mg sodium, 0mg cholesterol

Spicy Tofu

Although tofu tends to be bland in taste, when marinated in a spicy marinade, it readily absorbs the flavors. I like to serve it with a mixed green salad and Sesame Broccoli (page 304). This spicy dish also is delicious when cut into cubes and added to a soup or a savory stew.

4 SERVINGS

1 package (16 ounces) extra firm tofu
1 tablespoon Asian sesame oil
1 tablespoon soy sauce
1 teaspoon red wine vinegar
1 clove garlic, minced
¼ teaspoon ground coriander
¼ teaspoon ground turmeric
¼ teaspoon dried basil
¼ teaspoon dried marjoram leaves
¼ teaspoon dried red pepper flakes
¼ teaspoon coarse salt
¼ teaspoon freshly ground pepper

PLACE the tofu on a double thickness of paper towels and blot dry. Cut the tofu in half horizontally and then cut each piece in half (there should be 4 equal-size pieces). Set aside.

To make the Spicy Tofu Marinade, combine the rest of the ingredients in a nonreactive dish and blend well. Add the tofu and turn to coat all over. Cover, and refrigerate for several hours or overnight, turning the tofu at least once.

Preheat the oven to 375 degrees F. Lightly coat a rimmed baking sheet with a nonstick vegetable spray.

Remove the tofu from the marinade (discard the marinade). Place the tofu on the prepared baking sheet and bake for 20 to 25 minutes. Serve immediately.

EACH SERVING PROVIDES:

3g carbohydrates, 99 calories, 9g protein, 6g fat,
0g dietary fiber, 447mg sodium, 0mg cholesterol

(continues)

Tofu, sometimes called bean curd or soybean curd, is a high-protein soy food. It is made from dry soybeans that are soaked in water to soften and then are crushed. The crushed soybeans are ladled into boiling water and allowed to boil gently for about 10 minutes. This boiled mass of beans next is separated into pulp and soy milk. A coagulant, such as calcium sulfate or magnesium chloride, is added to the warm soy milk in order to separate it into curds and whey. Once separated, the curds float to the top and the whey remains on the bottom. Finally, the curds are gently removed and ladled into molds where they form into solid tofu blocks.

The two varieties of fresh tofu most commonly found in the supermarket are:

Firm or Chinese-Style Tofu: This dense and firm tofu is coarse-looking in appearance yet is very smooth when cooked. Due to its density, firm tofu works well in stir-fry dishes, soups, or grilling and also will tolerate being marinated for a long period of time. It also is higher in protein, calcium, and fat than the other varieties of tofu. Firm tofu is packaged with water in sealed plastic containers. Once opened, the water should be changed each day, refilling with enough fresh water to cover. Firm tofu always should be refrigerated.

Silken Tofu: Silken tofu has a creamy, custardlike texture and can be found in soft or firm varieties. It is more fragile than the firm tofu, so it is best to use it in soups or salads. It also can be pureed or made into sauces or mayonnaise. This variety of tofu will stand up to being baked, broiled, or sautéed, but it must be handled carefully. Silken tofu is packaged in water-filled tubs, aseptic brick packages, or vacuum-packed containers. Since it is ultrapasteurized, it has a long shelf life, but once opened, it should be refrigerated for up to four days.

Spinach and Ricotta Tart

Serve this fabulously rich and delicious crustless spinach tart to your fellow low-carbohydrate dieters and all their cravings will be instantly satisfied.

10 SERVINGS

1 tablespoon extra virgin
  olive oil
½ cup chopped yellow onion
1 large clove garlic, minced
1 box (10 ounces) frozen
  chopped spinach, defrosted
  and squeezed dry
16 ounces ricotta cheese

1 cup shredded Swiss cheese
4 eggs, lightly beaten
½ teaspoon coarse salt
½ teaspoon dried basil
⅛ teaspoon freshly ground
  pepper
⅛ teaspoon ground nutmeg

PREHEAT oven to 375 degrees F. Lightly coat a 9-inch quiche or pie pan with a nonstick vegetable spray Set aside.

Heat a medium skillet over medium heat for 2 minutes. Add the olive oil and swirl the pan to coat the bottom evenly. Add the onion and garlic and sauté for 2 minutes or until golden brown, stirring frequently.

Combine the onion mixture and the rest of the ingredients in a medium bowl and blend well. Spoon the spinach mixture into the prepared pan and bake for 40 minutes or until set in the center. Cool at least 10 minutes before serving.

To serve, cut the tart into wedges and place each one on a dinner plate.

EACH SERVING PROVIDES:
4g carbohydrates, 171 calories, 11g protein, 12g fat,
1g dietary fiber, 202mg sodium, 118mg cholesterol

Thai Marinated Portobello Mushrooms

Portobello mushrooms are exceptionally delicious when marinated in a Thai-infused potion. They readily absorb the flavors of this marinade and others you may wish to create. When braised, these giant mushrooms cook up almost like a steak. Thinly sliced, they are a vegetarian's dream come true. Serve with Green Beans with Hazelnuts (page 297).

4 SERVINGS

8 medium Portobello mushrooms, stems removed

1 recipe Thai Marinade (page 201)

4 to 6 tablespoons canola oil

Thai Dipping Sauce (page 201) (optional)

USE a damp paper towel to clean the Portobello mushrooms. Combine the mushrooms and Thai Marinade in a large resealable plastic bag and turn to coat all over. Seal the bag, and refrigerate for 2 hours, turning the mushrooms at least once.

Heat a large nonstick skillet over medium heat. Add 3 tablespoons canola oil and swirl the pan to coat the bottom evenly. Remove the Portobello mushrooms from the marinade (discard the marinade). Place half the mushrooms in the skillet and cook for 5 minutes on each side or until brown. Remove the mushrooms to a double thickness of paper towels to absorb any grease. Cook the remaining mushrooms in the skillet, adding additional canola oil, 1 tablespoon at a time, if necessary. Using a sharp knife, thinly slice the Portobello mushrooms on the diagonal, as you would a brisket or flank steak.

To serve, arrange the Portobello mushroom slices on each of four dinner plates. Serve with small bowls of Thai Dipping Sauce, if desired.

EACH SERVING PROVIDES:
13g carbohydrates, 216 calories, 9g protein, 17g fat,
8g dietary fiber, 822mg sodium, 0mg cholesterol

Tofu Curry

One of the key components of this hot curry sauce is red curry paste, which is a blend of chilis and spices. It is an essential ingredient used in Thai cooking. Curry pastes are identified as red, green, or yellow, and the color of each is dependent on the kind of chili it contains. Serve this recipe with Sautéed Zucchini (page 302).

4 SERVINGS

1 package (16 ounces) extra firm tofu
1½ cups unsweetened pure coconut milk
¼ cup natural peanut butter
2 tablespoons red curry paste*

1 teaspoon ground turmeric
¼ teaspoon curry powder
⅛ teaspoon coarse salt
1 red bell pepper, cut into julienne strips

PLACE the tofu on a double thickness of paper towels and blot dry. Cut the tofu into 1-inch cubes. Set aside.

To make the Curry Sauce, combine the coconut milk, peanut butter, curry paste, turmeric, curry, and salt in a large skillet over medium heat and blend well. Add the red pepper and blend. Bring to a simmer, stirring occasionally. Add the tofu and blend. Cook for 2 minutes or until heated through, stirring occasionally.

EACH SERVING PROVIDES:

13g carbohydrates, 378 calories, 15g protein, 32g fat,
4g dietary fiber, 171mg sodium, 0mg cholesterol

*Red curry paste is available in Asian food shops.

chapter eight

VERITABLE
VEGETABLES

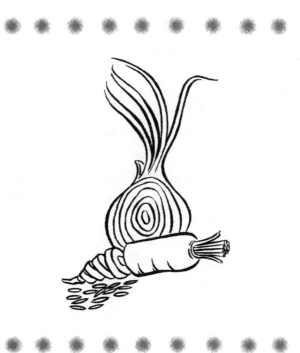

VEGETABLES

Asian Green Bean Stir-Fry

Asparagus Custard

Asparagus with Mustard Sauce

Asparagus with Orange Sauce

Balsamic Glazed Brussels Sprouts

Balsamic-Infused Cabbage

Broccoli with Garlic and Cheese

Brussels Sprouts with
    Cardamom

Brussels Sprouts with Mustard
    Sauce

Cauliflower Puree

Creamed Spinach

Greek Marinated Vegetable
    Kebabs

Green Bean Rice

Green Beans and Red Pepper

Green Beans with Buttered
    Almonds

Green Beans with Cheese and
    Cashews

Green Beans with Garlic and Red
    Pepper Flakes

Green Beans with Hazelnuts

Mushrooms with Parmesan
    Cheese

Mustard-Scented Green Beans

Roasted Asparagus

Sautéed Spinach with Garlic and
    Pine Nuts

Sautéed Zucchini

Savory Mushrooms

Sesame Broccoli

Spinach Custard

Steamed Broccoli with Lemon
    Butter Sauce

Szechwan Eggplant

Zesty Green Beans

Zucchini and Goat Cheese
    Gratin

Zucchini and Green Olive
    Medley

Zucchini Matchsticks

Zucchini Pasta

Zucchini Soufflé

Zucchini and Swiss Cheese
    Soufflé

U NFORTUNATELY, MANY OF OUR favorite vegetables, such as potatoes, carrots, and winter squash, are very high in carbohydrates. For this reason, they are not allowed on most low-carbohydrate diets. But I promise you, there really is life beyond French fried potatoes. Many other vegetables are allowed on this diet and, when prepared with the right herbs, spices, and other flavor-enhancing ingredients, can be transformed into mouth-watering offerings. The appeal of many of these garden delights can be heightened by simply combining them with a complementary cheese or by roasting them in the oven. What's more, many vegetable dishes can stand on their own as a hearty vegetarian meal. Should there be any leftovers, these same vegetable creations can be made into a zesty soup by simply pureeing them and adding the appropriate amount of broth, while others, combined with eggs, can be transformed into a savory vegetable omelet.

After you have had an opportunity to try many of the recipes found in this chapter, I hope you will agree with me that low-carbohydrate dieting and vegetables go hand in hand. But before embarking on this exciting adventure, I also would like to share delightful discoveries I made about two particular low-carbohydrate vegetables.

I found that by simply cutting zucchini into matchsticks or pasta-size strips and then sautéing, steaming, or boiling them, they could be readily substituted for pasta in many dishes. True, zucchini strips do not look or taste precisely like linguini, but, mama mia!, when you have a craving for pasta, this is the closest low-carbohydrate alternative around.

Another versatile vegetable is the green bean. How often does a recipe suggest serving a stir-fry or stew on a bed of rice? When green beans are very thinly sliced and cooked well, they make the perfect foil for rice. When prepared in this manner, they may not be white and fluffy, but they are a very tasty, colorful, and somewhat crunchy alternative.

If you are craving something rich and creamy, Cauliflower Puree or Creamed Spinach is certain to satisfy. Or, if you are in the mood for a hearty casserole, then Zucchini Soufflé has your name on it. So, what are you waiting for? With such a wide array of tempting vegetable dishes from which to choose, low-carbohydrate dieting will never be more rewarding and enjoyable.

Asian Green Bean Stir-Fry

Ginger, garlic, soy sauce, and sesame oil are a winning combination when you want to infuse green beans with the flavors of the Orient. They are also delicious served hot or cold, so you might consider doubling the recipe to ensure that you will have leftovers.

4 SERVINGS

6 tablespoons chicken broth
2 tablespoons soy sauce
2 teaspoons Asian sesame oil
1 pound green beans, trimmed
1 clove garlic, minced

1 tablespoon minced fresh
  ginger
1 teaspoon toasted sesame seeds
  (optional)

COMBINE the chicken broth and soy sauce in a small dish and blend well. Set aside.

Heat a large skillet over medium-high heat for 1 minute. Add the sesame oil and swirl the pan to coat the bottom evenly. Add the green beans and stir-fry for 5 minutes. Add the chicken stock mixture, garlic, and ginger and stir-fry for 1 minute. Cover the skillet and cook for 2 minutes. Remove the cover and continue to cook until there is no liquid remaining in the skillet. Sprinkle with sesame seeds, if desired.

EACH SERVING PROVIDES:
9g carbohydrates, 64 calories, 3g protein, 2g fat,
4g dietary fiber, 617mg sodium, 0mg cholesterol

Asparagus Custard

If you are not already an asparagus lover, this custard definitely will make you reconsider. This springtime vegetable delight is especially delicious when topped with Orange Sauce (page 280).

4 SERVINGS

1 pound asparagus, tough ends removed and cut into 2-inch lengths
2 tablespoons butter, at room temperature
4 eggs

⅔ cup freshly grated Parmesan cheese
1 tablespoon chopped fresh chives
½ teaspoon coarse salt
¼ teaspoon freshly ground pepper

PREHEAT the oven to 350 degrees F. Lightly coat a 1-quart baking dish with a nonstick vegetable spray. Set aside.

Bring salted water to a rolling boil in a medium saucepan. Add the asparagus and boil for 4 minutes. Drain well. Pat dry with paper towels.

Transfer the asparagus to the work bowl of a food processor fitted with a metal blade (or in a blender) and process until pureed. Add the butter and blend until incorporated. Add the remaining ingredients and process until smooth.

Spoon the asparagus mixture into the prepared baking dish. Bake for 35 to 40 minutes or until set in the center. Serve immediately.

EACH SERVING PROVIDES:
6g carbohydrates, 219 calories, 15g protein, 15g fat,
2g dietary fiber, 604mg sodium, 216mg cholesterol

Asparagus with Mustard Sauce

This delicious Mustard Sauce is a fabulous way to transform asparagus into an elegant dish. It also nicely enhances the flavor of broccoli, green beans, Brussels sprouts, or just about any of your favorite low-carbohydrate vegetables!

6 SERVINGS

¼ cup Dijon mustard
2 tablespoons red wine vinegar
1 teaspoon Splenda or other
   artificial sweetener

¼ teaspoon coarse salt
2 tablespoons canola oil
1¼ pounds asparagus spears,
   tough ends removed

To make the Mustard Sauce, combine the mustard, red wine vinegar, Splenda, and salt in a small bowl and blend well. Gradually whisk in the canola oil and beat until well blended. Set aside.

Place the asparagus in a vegetable steamer filled with about 2 inches of boiling water. Steam for 5 to 7 minutes or until crisp-tender. Or, blanch the asparagus in boiling water for 1 to 2 minutes. Drain well. Pat dry with paper towels.

To serve, place the asparagus spears on each of six plates, dividing evenly. Spoon some Mustard Sauce over each serving.

EACH SERVING PROVIDES:
6g carbohydrates, 75 calories, 3g protein, 6g fat,
2g dietary fiber, 333mg sodium, 0mg cholesterol

Asparagus with Orange Sauce

Asparagus is a wonderful vegetable that is delicious when served simply steamed or blanched. Spooning a touch of richly flavored Orange Sauce over these green delights, however, elevates them to a new dimension.

4 SERVINGS

¼ cup butter
¼ cup fresh orange juice
1 tablespoon finely grated
   orange rind

1 pound fresh asparagus spears,
   tough ends removed

To make the Orange Sauce, combine the butter, orange juice, and orange rind in a small saucepan over medium-high heat. Cook for 4 to 5 minutes or just until the sauce thickens.

Bring salted water to a rolling boil in a large skillet. Add the asparagus and blanch for 1 to 2 minutes or just until crisp-tender. Transfer the asparagus to a colander and immediately rinse with cold water. Drain well. Pat dry with paper towels.

To serve, place the asparagus spears on each of four dinner plates, dividing evenly. Drizzle some Orange Sauce over each serving.

EACH SERVING PROVIDES:
7g carbohydrates, 136 calories, 3g protein, 12g fat,
3g dietary fiber, 4mg sodium, 31mg cholesterol

Balsamic Glazed Brussels Sprouts

If Brussels sprouts are not high on your list of favorite vegetables, you will quickly change your mind after one taste of these bite-size gems.

4 SERVINGS

1 pound Brussels sprouts
2 tablespoons extra virgin
   olive oil
¼ cup thinly sliced yellow onion
1 large clove garlic, thinly sliced

2 tablespoons balsamic vinegar
¼ teaspoon coarse salt
¼ teaspoon freshly ground
   pepper

CUT the ends off the Brussels sprouts and remove any dead leaves. Using a sharp knife, cut an "×" on the bottom of each. (This method brings the heat to the centers of the Brussels sprouts.)

Bring salted water to a rolling boil in a medium saucepan. Add the Brussels sprouts and boil for 5 minutes. Transfer the Brussels sprouts to a colander and drain well.

Heat a large skillet over medium heat for 2 minutes. Add the olive oil and swirl the pan to coat the bottom evenly. Add the onion and garlic and sauté for 2 to 3 minutes or until the onion is tender, stirring frequently. Add the Brussels sprouts and sauté for 3 to 4 minutes or until heated through, stirring occasionally. Add the balsamic vinegar and toss the Brussels sprouts until they are well coated. Season with salt and pepper and gently toss.

EACH SERVING PROVIDES:

12g carbohydrates, 121 calories, 4g protein, 7g fat,
4g dietary fiber, 148mg sodium, 0mg cholesterol

Balsamic-Infused Cabbage

It is not an easy task to get my family to eat cabbage, but this is one dish they adore. Of course, I believe anything flavored with balsamic vinegar has to taste great.

4 SERVINGS

½ cup diced raw bacon
¼ cup balsamic vinegar
4 cups thinly sliced cabbage
1 cup cold water

½ teaspoon coarse salt
½ teaspoon freshly ground
   pepper

PLACE a large nonstick skillet over medium heat for 1 minute. Add the bacon and sauté for 4 to 5 minutes or until crisp, stirring occasionally. Add the balsamic vinegar and cook until most of the liquid has evaporated. Add the cabbage and water and bring to a boil over medium-high heat. Cover, and cook over medium-low heat for 10 minutes or until the cabbage is tender. Using a slotted spoon, transfer the cabbage to a serving dish. Season with salt and pepper and lightly blend. Serve immediately.

EACH SERVING PROVIDES:

6g carbohydrates, 82 calories, 4g protein, 5g fat,
2g dietary fiber, 457mg sodium, 8mg cholesterol

Broccoli with Garlic and Cheese

If you are a confirmed broccoli hater, you will surrender after one taste of garlic-flavored broccoli encased in a delicate cheese.

4 SERVINGS

1 pound broccoli florets	2 cloves garlic, minced
2 tablespoons extra virgin olive oil	¼ cup freshly grated Romano cheese

PLACE the broccoli in a vegetable steamer filled with about 2 inches of boiling water. Steam for 2 minutes. Drain well.

Heat a large nonstick skillet over medium heat for 2 minutes. Add the olive oil and swirl the pan to coat the bottom evenly. Add the garlic and sauté for 1 minute or until fragrant. Add the broccoli and sauté for 3 to 4 minutes or until heated through, stirring frequently. Remove the skillet from the heat. Sprinkle the cheese over the broccoli and toss lightly. Season with salt and pepper, if desired.

EACH SERVING PROVIDES:
7g carbohydrates, 121 calories, 5g protein, 9g fat,
3g dietary fiber, 106mg sodium, 7mg cholesterol

Brussels Sprouts with Cardamom

Cardamom is a spice similar in taste to ginger. What sets it apart, however, is the hint of lemony flavor it imparts to foods. This quality makes it the ideal spice to combine with Brussels sprouts.

4 SERVINGS

4 cardamom pods (or ¼ tea-
    spoon ground cardamom)
1 pound Brussels sprouts
2 tablespoons butter

½ tablespoon finely grated
    orange peel
⅛ teaspoon salt

PLACE the cardamom pods in a spice grinder and grind into a powder. Set aside.

Cut the ends off the Brussels sprouts and remove any dead leaves. Using a sharp knife, cut an "×" on the bottom of each. (This method brings the heat to the centers of the Brussels sprouts.)

Place the Brussels sprouts in a vegetable steamer filled with about 2 inches of boiling water. Steam for 15 minutes or until fork tender. (It may be necessary to add additional water during the steaming process.) Drain well.

Melt the butter in a medium saucepan over medium heat. Add the Brussels sprouts, orange peel, and cardamom and cook for 1 to 2 minutes or until heated through, stirring frequently. Season with salt.

EACH SERVING PROVIDES:

10g carbohydrates, 101 calories, 4g protein, 6g fat,
4g dietary fiber, 102mg sodium, 16mg cholesterol

ABOUT BRUSSELS SPROUTS

Brussels sprouts are a member of the cruciferous family and therefore are related to cabbage and cauliflower. When first sprouting, the stem sends up a long shoot with the sprouts forming close to the ground. As they mature, others appear higher up on the stalk. Each one looks like a small head of cabbage, measuring from ½ to 1 inch in diameter. Not surprisingly, Brussels sprouts were first cultivated in Brussels. These nutritional wonders, available from September through January, are an excellent source of vitamins A and C.

When choosing Brussels sprouts, look for ones that are dark green, firm, and tightly formed. Select those with smaller heads for their more delicate flavor. Avoid any with yellow or wilted leaves. Store the Brussels sprouts in an airtight plastic bag in the refrigerator and wash them just before using them.

Brussels Sprouts with Mustard Sauce

Brussels sprouts are magically transformed into a temptingly delicious vegetable by simply adding this piquant sauce. In fact, this sauce could perform this same feat with broccoli, green beans, or cauliflower.

4 SERVINGS

2 tablespoons Dijon mustard
2 teaspoons soy sauce
1 teaspoon Asian sesame oil
1 pound Brussels sprouts

1 tablespoon canola oil
½ cup thinly sliced green
  onions

To make the Mustard Sauce, combine the mustard, soy sauce, and sesame oil in a small dish and blend well. Set aside.

Cut the ends off the Brussels sprouts and remove any dead leaves. Using a sharp knife, cut an "×" on the bottom of each. (This method brings the heat to the centers of the Brussels sprouts.)

Place the Brussels sprouts in a vegetable steamer filled with about 2 inches of boiling water. Steam for 15 minutes or until fork tender. (It may be necessary to add water during the steaming process.) Drain well.

Place a large skillet over medium-high heat for 1 minute. Add the canola oil and swirl the pan to coat the bottom evenly. Add the green onions and stir-fry for 2 minutes. Add the Brussels sprouts and stir-fry for 1 to 2 minutes or until heated through. Spoon the Mustard Sauce over the Brussels sprouts and lightly toss. Serve immediately.

EACH SERVING PROVIDES:
12g carbohydrates, 104 calories, 5g protein, 6g fat,
5g dietary fiber, 391mg sodium, 0mg cholesterol

Cauliflower Puree

This delicious dish is dedicated to all cauliflower devotees. Rich and creamy, its flavor and color make it the perfect accompaniment for most entrées.

4 SERVINGS

1 pound cauliflower, broken into small florets

¼ cup freshly grated Parmesan cheese

¼ cup whipping cream

1 tablespoon butter, at room temperature

¼ teaspoon coarse salt

⅛ teaspoon freshly grated pepper

PLACE the cauliflower in a vegetable steamer filled with about 2 inches of boiling water. Steam for 18 to 20 minutes or until fork tender. (It may be necessary to add additional water during the steaming process.) Drain well.

Place the cauliflower in the work bowl of a food processor fitted with a metal blade (or in a blender) and process until pureed. Add the rest of the ingredients and pulse to lightly blend. Taste for seasoning. (The cauliflower puree can be prepared a day ahead. Transfer the cauliflower to a covered dish and refrigerate. Reheat over low heat before serving.)

EACH SERVING PROVIDES:

7g carbohydrates, 134 calories, 5g protein, 11g fat,
3g dietary fiber, 274mg sodium, 33mg cholesterol

ABOUT CAULIFLOWER

Cauliflower originated in Asia, but the cauliflower we know today was perfected in Italy. It is a member of the cruciferous family. It has a large head made up of edible, creamy white, clustered, juicy flowers surrounded by large green leaves.

When choosing cauliflower, look for firm heads with creamy white clusters and void of any spots or bruises that indicate it may not be fresh. Wash the cauliflower well and, when dry, store in a perforated plastic bag in the refrigerator.

Creamed Spinach

How many of us grew up hearing "Eat your spinach"? Well, this is one spinach dish for which your family won't require any prompting. Instead, you're likely to hear, "More, please." Slightly garlicky and richly creamy, this flavorful creation is irresistible.

4 SERVINGS

1 tablespoon extra virgin olive oil

1 large clove garlic, minced

1 pound prewashed spinach

½ cup whipping cream

¼ teaspoon coarse salt

¼ teaspoon freshly ground pepper

HEAT a large skillet over high heat for 1 minute. Add the olive oil and garlic and swirl the pan to coat the bottom evenly with the oil. Add the spinach and stir-fry for 1 to 2 minutes or until the spinach begins to wilt. Transfer the spinach to a towel and roll up the towel to blot up the excess moisture. Coarsely chop the spinach, if desired.

Heat the whipping cream in the same skillet over high heat for 2 minutes or until it begins to thicken. Add the spinach and blend well. Season with salt and pepper. Cook until heated through, stirring frequently. Serve immediately.

EACH SERVING PROVIDES:

5g carbohydrates, 161 calories, 4g protein, 15g fat,
3g dietary fiber, 219mg sodium, 41mg cholesterol

Greek Marinated Vegetable Kebabs

I can't think of a better accompaniment to serve with Greek Chicken (page 197) than these flavorful vegetable kebabs. You can substitute any of your favorite low-carbohydrate vegetables for the ones I suggested—you can't go wrong with this recipe.

4 SERVINGS

1 recipe Greek Vinaigrette (page 142)

1 large red bell pepper, cut into 1-inch cubes

1 small yellow onion, peeled and cut into 8 wedges

2 zucchini, cut into ½-inch-thick rounds

1 eggplant, cut into 1½-inch cubes

8 cherry tomatoes

PLACE 8- to 10-inch wooden skewers in a pan of water and allow them to soak for at least 30 minutes or more.

Place the Greek Vinaigrette in a large resealable plastic bag. Add the vegetables and turn to coat all over. Seal the bag, and refrigerate for up to 1 hour.

When ready to grill, remove the vegetables from the Greek Vinaigrette (reserve the vinaigrette) and thread them onto the skewers. It is best to thread the vegetables on double-pronged skewers or two wooden skewers that are parallel to each other, about 1 inch apart. This will prevent the vegetables from spinning around when the skewer is turned, making it easier to cook them evenly on both sides. Place the skewers on a grill coated with a nonstick vegetable spray over medium-hot coals. Brush generously with the reserved Greek Vinaigrette. Cover the grill and cook for 4 to 5 minutes on each side or until the vegetables are lightly charred.

EACH SERVING PROVIDES:

19g carbohydrates, 257 calories, 3g protein, 20g fat, 6g dietary fiber, 174mg sodium, 0mg cholesterol

Green Bean Rice

There are many wonderful stir-fries or stews begging to be paired with rice. Since rice is taboo on many low-carbohydrate diets, I came up with this idea to slice green beans thinly and cook them long enough to make them tender, and presto, you have a substitute for rice.

4 SERVINGS

1 pound green beans, trimmed
Salt

STACK several green beans together, and patiently cut them into very thin slices, about $\frac{1}{8}$- to $\frac{1}{4}$-inch thick.

Bring salted water to a rolling boil in a large saucepan over high heat. Add the green beans and cook for 6 to 7 minutes or until fork tender. Transfer the green beans to a colander and drain well. Pat dry with paper towels.

EACH SERVING PROVIDES:

8g carbohydrates, 35 calories, 2g protein, 0g fat,

4g dietary fiber, 7mg sodium, 0mg cholesterol

Green Beans and Red Pepper

This colorful vegetable combo would add a festive touch to an extravagant holiday buffet or a simple family dinner. With the addition of balsamic vinegar, the beans acquire a distinctively robust flavor as well as a rich color. If you prefer less color, try substituting with white balsamic vinegar—it remains as delicious as ever.

6 SERVINGS

1½ pounds green beans, trimmed

2 tablespoons extra virgin olive oil

1 red bell pepper, cut into ¼-inch-wide strips

2 cloves garlic, minced

¼ cup balsamic vinegar

½ teaspoon coarse salt

½ teaspoon freshly ground pepper

BRING salted water to a rolling boil in a large saucepan. Add the green beans and boil for 5 to 6 minutes or until crisp-tender. Transfer the green beans to a colander and rinse with cold water. Drain well. Pat dry with paper towels. (The green beans can be cooked in the morning. Place them in a covered container and refrigerate until ready to use.)

Heat a large skillet over medium heat for 2 minutes. Add the olive oil and swirl the pan to coat the bottom evenly. Add the red pepper and garlic and sauté for 3 minutes or until the red peppers are crisp-tender. Add the green beans, balsamic vinegar, salt, and pepper and stir-fry until the beans are heated through.

EACH SERVING PROVIDES:
11g carbohydrates, 91 calories, 2g protein, 5g fat,
4g dietary fiber, 167mg sodium, 0mg cholesterol

Green Beans with Buttered Almonds

Pairing green beans and buttered almonds provides a nice contrast in flavors, texture, and color. You also can make this delectable dish with asparagus or broccoli.

4 SERVINGS

1 pound green beans, trimmed
3 tablespoons butter
½ cup sliced almonds

¼ teaspoon coarse salt
¼ teaspoon freshly ground
  pepper

BRING salted water to a rolling boil in a large saucepan over high heat. Add the green beans and cook for 5 to 6 minutes or until crisp-tender. Transfer the green beans to a colander and rinse with cold water. Pat dry with paper towels. (The green beans can be cooked in the morning. Place them in a covered container and refrigerate until ready to use.)

Melt the butter in a large skillet over medium heat. Add the almonds, salt, and pepper and sauté for 2 minutes, stirring frequently. Add the green beans and sauté for 2 minutes or until heated through, stirring constantly.

EACH SERVING PROVIDES:

10g carbohydrates, 183 calories, 5g protein, 15g fat,
5g dietary fiber, 126mg sodium, 23mg cholesterol

ABOUT BEANS

There is a wide variety of summer beans that comes in an assortment of sizes, colors, and shapes. Pole beans refer to the variety of beans that grows on a pole, while bush beans grow close to the ground. Pole beans are easily recognizable by their long and plump appearance. Haricots verts is a prime example of a bush bean. This French green bean is very skinny and exceptionally tender.

When choosing beans, look for those that are firm and with good color. Wash the beans well and, when dry, place them in an airtight plastic bag in the refrigerator for a few days.

Green Beans with Cheese and Cashews

Green beans never tasted better. Although easy to prepare, this dish is elegant enough to be served at a festive dinner.

4 SERVINGS

1 pound green beans, trimmed
3 tablespoons butter
2 teaspoons curry powder
½ cup thinly sliced yellow
  onions

¼ cup unsalted roasted cashews
1 cup shredded sharp Cheddar
  cheese

BRING salted water to a rolling boil in a large saucepan over high heat. Add the green beans and cook for 3 minutes. Transfer the green beans to a colander and rinse with cold water. Pat dry with paper towels. (The green beans can be cooked in the morning. Place them in a covered container and refrigerate until ready to use.)

Melt the butter in a large skillet over moderate heat. Add the curry and cook for 1 minute or until fragrant, stirring frequently. Add the onion, cashews, and green beans and cook, stirring occasionally, for about 5 minutes or until the green beans are fork tender. Sprinkle the Cheddar cheese over the green beans. Cover for 1 minute or until the cheese melts. Lightly blend and serve immediately.

EACH SERVING PROVIDES:
13g carbohydrates, 255 calories, 13g protein, 18g fat,
5g dietary fiber, 207mg sodium, 40mg cholesterol

Green Beans with Garlic and Red Pepper Flakes

Green beans take on an entirely new taste when accented with garlic. I often like to substitute broccoli, broccoli rabe, or cauliflower for a change—let your imagination take wing.

4 SERVINGS

1 pound green beans, trimmed
2 tablespoons extra virgin
   olive oil

1 large clove garlic, coarsely
   chopped
$\frac{1}{4}$ teaspoon dried red pepper
   flakes

BRING salted water to a rolling boil in a large saucepan. Add the green beans and cook for 5 to 6 minutes or until crisp-tender. Transfer the green beans to a colander and rinse with cold water. Drain well. Pat dry with paper towels.

Heat a large skillet over medium heat for 2 minutes. Add the olive oil and swirl the pan to coat the bottom evenly. Add the garlic and red pepper flakes and cook for 1 minute or until fragrant. Add the green beans and cook until heated through, stirring constantly.

EACH SERVING PROVIDES:
8g carbohydrates, 100 calories, 2g protein, 7g fat,
4g dietary fiber, 7mg sodium, 0mg cholesterol

Green Beans with Hazelnuts

The hazelnuts provide just enough flavor, crunch, and color to transform green beans into an extraordinary dish. I usually double the recipe so I can have leftovers the next day.

4 SERVINGS

1 pound green beans, trimmed
2 tablespoons butter
1 shallot, minced
½ teaspoon coarse salt

¼ teaspoon freshly ground pepper
¼ cup toasted hazelnuts, coarsely chopped*

BRING salted water to a rolling boil in a large saucepan. Add the green beans and cook for 5 to 6 minutes or until crisp-tender. Transfer the green beans to a colander and rinse with cold water. Drain well. Pat dry with paper towels. (The green beans can be cooked in the morning. Place them in a covered container and refrigerate until ready to use.)

Melt the butter in a large skillet over medium heat. Add the shallot, salt, and pepper and cook for 4 minutes, stirring occasionally. Add the green beans and hazelnuts and cook until heated through, stirring constantly.

EACH SERVING PROVIDES:

11g carbohydrates, 124 calories, 3g protein, 9g fat,
5g dietary fiber, 244mg sodium, 16mg cholesterol

*To toast hazelnuts: Preheat the oven to 350 degrees F, spread the hazelnuts in a single layer in a shallow pan, and bake for 10 minutes or until fragrant.

Mushrooms with Parmesan Cheese

This robust side dish features mushrooms and Parmesan cheese. Fresh herbs and spices deepen the flavor of this hearty vegetable combination.

4 SERVINGS

1 pound fresh button mushrooms, stems removed
1 tablespoon cold water
3 tablespoons freshly grated Parmesan cheese
1 tablespoon chopped fresh parsley (or Italian leaf parsley)
1 large clove garlic, minced
½ teaspoon coarse salt
½ teaspoon dried oregano leaves
¼ teaspoon freshly ground pepper
¼ teaspoon fresh thyme leaves (or ¼ teaspoon dried thyme leaves)
3 tablespoons extra virgin olive oil

PREHEAT oven to 350 degrees F. Place the mushrooms, stem side up, in a baking dish large enough to hold them in a single layer. Pour the water around the mushrooms.

Combine the cheese, parsley, garlic, salt, oregano, pepper, and thyme in a small bowl and blend well. Sprinkle the cheese mixture over the mushrooms and drizzle with olive oil. Bake for 15 minutes or until golden brown.

EACH SERVING PROVIDES:
6g carbohydrates, 147 calories, 4g protein, 12g fat,
2g dietary fiber, 328mg sodium, 4mg cholesterol

Mustard-Scented Green Beans

Dijon mustard adds a zesty flavor to green beans as well as to many of your other favorite low-carbohydrate vegetables.

4 SERVINGS

2 tablespoons Dijon mustard
2 teaspoons extra virgin
   olive oil
⅛ teaspoon coarse salt

⅛ teaspoon freshly ground
   pepper
1 pound green beans, trimmed

COMBINE the mustard, olive oil, salt, and pepper in a small bowl until well blended. Set aside.

Bring salted water to a rolling boil in a large saucepan. Add the green beans and boil for 6 to 7 minutes or until fork tender. Transfer the green beans to a colander and drain well.

Place the green beans in a serving bowl. Add the Dijon mustard mixture and blend well.

EACH SERVING PROVIDES:

9g carbohydrates, 66 calories, 3g protein, 3g fat,

4g dietary fiber, 255mg sodium, 0mg cholesterol

Roasted Asparagus

Once you have roasted asparagus this way, you will never want to have it any other way. The spears remain crisp yet the roasting enhances their unique flavor.

4 SERVINGS

1 to 2 tablespoons extra virgin
  olive oil
½ teaspoon coarse salt
½ teaspoon freshly ground
  pepper

1 pound medium to jumbo
  asparagus spears, tough
  ends removed
Freshly shaved Parmesan cheese
  (optional)

PREHEAT oven to 450 degrees F. Combine the olive oil, salt, and pepper in a large resealable plastic bag. Add the asparagus and turn to coat all over.

Place the asparagus in a single layer in a shallow pan. Bake for 10 to 15 minutes or just until fork tender. For an added touch, sprinkle freshly shaved Parmesan cheese over the hot asparagus.

EACH SERVING PROVIDES:
5g carbohydrates, 58 calories, 3g protein, 4g fat,
2g dietary fiber, 238mg sodium, 0mg cholesterol

Sautéed Spinach with Garlic and Pine Nuts

Spinach and garlic sautéed together make a fabulously tasty vegetable, but when toasted pine nuts are added, this dish becomes even more richly satisfying. It is the perfect accompaniment to a savory meat or poultry entrée.

4 SERVINGS

1 pound prewashed spinach
1 tablespoon extra virgin olive oil
1 large clove garlic, minced

¼ teaspoon coarse salt
⅛ teaspoon freshly ground pepper
¼ cup toasted pine nuts*

BRING one cup water to a boil in a large skillet over high heat. Add the spinach and cook, covered, over low heat for 4 minutes. Transfer the spinach to a colander and drain well. When the spinach is cool enough to handle, place it in a towel and squeeze out as much moisture as possible. Chop it finely. (The spinach can be prepared a day ahead. Place it in a covered container and refrigerate.)

Heat a large skillet over low heat for 2 minutes. Add the olive oil and swirl the pan to coat the bottom evenly. Add the garlic and cook for 1 minute or until fragrant, stirring frequently. Season with salt and pepper. Add the spinach and blend well. Cook until heated through. Add the pine nuts and blend.

EACH SERVING PROVIDES:

5g carbohydrates, 106 calories, 5g protein, 8g fat,
3g dietary fiber, 208mg sodium, 0mg cholesterol

*To toast pine nuts: Preheat the oven to 350 degrees F, place the pine nuts in a single layer in a shallow pan, and bake for 10 minutes or until golden brown.

Sautéed Zucchini

This vegetable is an example of how easy it is to create a vegetable with enough seasonings and herbs to instantly create a culinary delight. If you prefer to omit the butter, simply add an extra tablespoon of olive oil.

4 SERVINGS

1 tablespoon extra virgin
   olive oil
1 tablespoon butter
1½ pounds zucchini, cut into
   julienne strips
1 large clove garlic, minced

1 tablespoon chopped fresh
   parsley
½ teaspoon coarse salt
½ teaspoon freshly ground
   pepper
1 tablespoon fresh lemon juice

HEAT the olive oil and butter in a large skillet over medium-high heat until the butter melts. Add the zucchini and sauté for 5 to 10 minutes or until just beginning to brown, stirring frequently. Add the garlic, parsley, salt, and pepper and blend well. Cook for 1 to 2 minutes or until the garlic becomes fragrant. Squeeze the lemon juice over the zucchini, if desired. Serve immediately.

EACH SERVING PROVIDES:
6g carbohydrates, 84 calories, 2g protein, 7g fat,
2g dietary fiber, 242mg sodium, 8mg cholesterol

Savory Mushrooms

Once you have tasted these mushrooms, you will be dreaming up new ways to use them—if there are any left. The mushrooms can be added to an omelet, spooned on top of a savory steak, or added to a soup.

3 TO 4 SERVINGS

3 tablespoons extra virgin olive oil
1 large clove garlic, minced
½ teaspoon coarse salt
¼ teaspoon freshly ground pepper

1 pound assorted fresh button or wild mushrooms (such as morels, chanterelles, shiitakes, Portobellos, or oyster), thinly sliced
3 tablespoons chopped fresh parsley

COMBINE 1 tablespoon olive oil, garlic, salt, and pepper in a large re-sealable plastic bag and blend. Add the mushrooms and turn to coat all over.

Heat a large skillet over medium heat for 2 minutes. Add 2 tablespoons olive oil and swirl the pan to coat the bottom evenly. Add the mushrooms and sauté for 8 to 10 minutes or until golden brown, stirring frequently. Season with salt and pepper and blend well. Add the parsley and lightly blend.

EACH SERVING PROVIDES:
8g carbohydrates, 167 calories, 3g protein, 15g fat,
2g dietary fiber, 322mg sodium, 0mg cholesterol

Sesame Broccoli

Sesame broccoli is an example of how you can effortlessly create a memorable side dish. Accented with the flavors of the Orient, this ordinary vegetable becomes an enticing accompaniment for any meal.

4 SERVINGS

1 pound broccoli florets
1 tablespoon rice vinegar
1 tablespoon soy sauce
1 tablespoon toasted sesame
  seeds*

½ tablespoon canola oil
1 teaspoon Splenda or other
  artificial sweetener

PLACE the broccoli in a vegetable steamer filled with about 2 inches of boiling water. Steam for 3 minutes. Drain well. Pat dry with paper towels.

Meanwhile, bring the other ingredients to a boil in a small saucepan over medium heat, stirring occasionally.

Place the broccoli in a serving dish. Pour the rice vinegar mixture over the broccoli and gently blend. Serve immediately.

EACH SERVING PROVIDES:
7g carbohydrates, 61 calories, 4g protein, 3g fat,
4g dietary fiber, 289mg sodium, 0mg cholesterol

*To toast sesame seeds: Preheat the oven to 350 degrees F, place the sesame seeds in a single layer in a shallow pan, and bake for 10 minutes or until golden.

Spinach Custard

Other than having to cook and squeeze dry the spinach, this is a deliciously easy way to enjoy this wonderful vegetable. It can be served as an accompaniment to a meal or even served as a first course when garnished with a Roasted Red Pepper Hollandaise Sauce. You also can substitute cauliflower, broccoli, or asparagus for the spinach.

4 SERVINGS

2 packages (10 ounces each) prewashed spinach

1 cup 2 percent milk, hot

2 tablespoons butter, at room temperature

2 tablespoons extra virgin olive oil

½ cup finely chopped yellow onion

¼ teaspoon coarse salt

¼ teaspoon freshly ground pepper

⅛ teaspoon ground nutmeg

5 eggs, beaten

½ cup shredded Swiss cheese

PREHEAT oven to 325 degrees F. Lightly coat a 5-cup ring mold or soufflé dish with a nonstick vegetable spray. Line the bottom with parchment or waxed paper and lightly coat with the spray again.

Bring 1 cup water to a boil in a large skillet over high heat. Add the spinach. Cover, and cook over low heat for 4 minutes. Transfer the spinach to a colander and drain well. When the spinach is cool enough to handle, place it in a towel and squeeze out as much moisture as possible. Chop the spinach coarsely. (The spinach can be prepared a day ahead. Place it in a covered container and refrigerate.)

Combine the hot milk and butter in a small pitcher and blend well. Set aside.

(continues)

Heat a large saucepan over medium heat for 2 minutes. Add the olive oil and swirl the pan to coat the bottom evenly. Add the onion and sauté for 4 minutes, stirring occasionally. Add the spinach, salt, pepper, and nutmeg and blend well. Add the milk mixture, eggs, and cheese and blend well. Spoon the mixture into the prepared mold.

Place the mold in a larger pan and put in the oven. Pour enough hot water into the pan to come halfway up the sides of the mold. Bake for 30 to 40 minutes or until a knife comes out clean when inserted in the center of the custard. Cool for at least 5 minutes.

To serve, run a knife along the sides of the custard and invert onto a serving dish; remove the paper. Serve immediately.

VARIATION: To make Roasted Red Pepper Hollandaise Sauce: Preheat the broiler and place two red peppers on a baking sheet lined with aluminum foil. Broil, turning the peppers as the skin blackens, for 20 to 25 minutes or until the skins are charred all over. Once the peppers are roasted, place them in a resealable plastic bag, seal, and allow them to steam for 15 to 20 minutes. When the peppers are cool enough to handle, peel away the skin and remove the tops and seeds. (Do not rinse the peppers.)

Place the red peppers in the work bowl of a food processor fitted with a metal blade (or in a blender) and process until pureed. Set aside.

In the clean work bowl of a food processor, combine four egg yolks, 1½ tablespoons fresh lemon juice, ¼ teaspoon coarse salt, and ⅛ teaspoon freshly ground pepper and process until blended. Add 2 tablespoons melted butter in a slow, steady stream and process until smooth. Add the pureed red peppers and blend.

EACH SERVING PROVIDES:
11g carbohydrates, 316 calories, 17g protein, 24g fat,
4g dietary fiber, 366mg sodium, 266mg cholesterol

Steamed Broccoli with Lemon Butter Sauce

Broccoli is a hardy vegetable that sparkles when accented with a lemon-flavored butter sauce. Try this sauce on some of your other favorite low-carbohydrate vegetables, such as asparagus or green beans.

4 SERVINGS

1 pound broccoli florets	4 drops Tabasco sauce or
2 tablespoons butter	favorite hot pepper sauce
2 tablespoons fresh lemon juice	½ tablespoon chopped fresh
⅛ teaspoon coarse salt	parsley

PLACE the broccoli in a vegetable steamer filled with about 2 inches of boiling water. Steam for 2 minutes. Drain well.

To make the Lemon Butter Sauce, melt the butter in a small saucepan over medium heat. Add the lemon juice, salt, and hot pepper sauce and blend well. Add the parsley and blend.

To serve, spoon some Lemon Butter Sauce over each serving of broccoli.

EACH SERVING PROVIDES:

7g carbohydrates, 85 calories, 3g protein, 6g fat,
3g dietary fiber, 92mg sodium, 16mg cholesterol

Szechwan Eggplant

Years ago, I took cooking lessons from a Chinese woman who offered classes in her home. This spicy dish was rated one of the favorites among the other students. The only ingredient you may not have readily available in your pantry is hot bean paste. I could only find hot bean sauce, which worked equally well. Either product may be available in most Asian food stores.

4 SERVINGS

2 medium eggplants (¾ pound each), trimmed
1 tablespoon canola oil
1 green onion, thinly sliced (optional)

Sauce #1
2 tablespoons soy sauce
1 tablespoon chopped garlic
1 tablespoon Splenda or other artificial sweetener

½ tablespoon chopped fresh ginger
½ tablespoon hot bean paste (or hot bean sauce)

Sauce #2
½ tablespoon Asian sesame oil
½ teaspoon white distilled vinegar

To make Sauce #1, combine all the ingredients in a small dish and blend well. Set aside.

To make Sauce #2, combine the sesame oil and vinegar in a small dish and set aside.

Cut the eggplant into finger-length strips, approximately 3 × ½ × ½ inches (it does not have to be exact).

Bring water to a rolling boil in a large saucepan. Add the eggplant and cook just until the water returns to a rolling boil. Transfer the eggplant to a colander and rinse with cold water. Drain well. Pat dry with paper towels.

Heat a large skillet over medium heat for 2 minutes. Add the canola oil and swirl the pan to coat the bottom evenly. Add Sauce #1 and the eggplant and stir-fry for 1 minute. Add Sauce #2 and stir-fry until heated through. Garnish each serving with green onion slices, if desired.

EACH SERVING PROVIDES:

17g carbohydrates, 120 calories, 3g protein, 6g fat,

5g dietary fiber, 527mg sodium, 0mg cholesterol

Zesty Green Beans

This green bean ensemble illustrates how easy it is to create an accompaniment, brimming with flavors, by simply combining a few basic ingredients.

4 SERVINGS

1 pound green beans, trimmed
2 tablespoons butter
½ cup chopped yellow onion
¼ teaspoon coarse salt

¼ teaspoon freshly ground
  pepper
½ teaspoon white wine vinegar

BRING salted water to a rolling boil in a large saucepan. Add the green beans and boil for 5 to 6 minutes or just until crisp-tender. Transfer the green beans to a colander and rinse with cold water. Drain well. Pat dry with paper towels.

In the same saucepan, melt the butter over medium-low heat. Add the onion and sauté for 4 minutes. Add the green beans, salt, and pepper and cook until heated through, stirring constantly. Add the vinegar and blend well.

EACH SERVING PROVIDES:
10g carbohydrates, 94 calories, 2g protein, 6g fat,
4g dietary fiber, 126mg sodium, 16mg cholesterol

Zucchini and Goat Cheese Gratin

The number of steps it takes to create this recipe is well worth the effort. It is a heavenly combination of zucchini and goat cheese that melds together to create a dish that is certain to impress your family and friends.

4 SERVINGS

1½ pounds zucchini, cut into ¼-inch-thick rounds

2 tablespoons extra virgin olive oil

½ cup thinly sliced yellow onion

½ teaspoon coarse salt

½ teaspoon freshly ground pepper

5 ounces goat cheese, such as Chèvre or Montrachet

⅓ cup whipping cream

3 tablespoons freshly grated Parmesan cheese

PREHEAT oven to 350 degrees F. Bring salted water to a rolling boil in a medium saucepan. Add the zucchini and boil for 2 minutes. Transfer the zucchini to a colander and drain well. Pat dry with paper towels. Set aside.

Heat a medium skillet over medium heat for 2 minutes. Add the olive oil and swirl the pan to coat the bottom evenly. Add the onion and sauté for 8 to 10 minutes or until translucent, stirring occasionally.

Lightly coat a 2-quart baking dish with a nonstick vegetable spray. Make a layer of one-third of the zucchini in the dish. Season lightly with some of the salt and pepper. Spread half the onion over the zucchini and season lightly with some of the salt and pepper. Repeat the layers, ending with the zucchini on top.

(continues)

Combine the goat cheese and whipping cream in a small saucepan over medium heat. Cook for 3 to 4 minutes or until the mixture is smooth and creamy, stirring occasionally. Spread this mixture over the zucchini and sprinkle Parmesan cheese on top. Bake for 40 minutes.

EACH SERVING PROVIDES:

7g carbohydrates, 278 calories, 11g protein, 23g fat,
2g dietary fiber, 466mg sodium, 47mg cholesterol

Zucchini and Green Olive Medley

This delicious medley of zucchini and olives makes the perfect accompaniment to a beef or chicken dish. Any leftover vegetables can be combined with eggs, cheese, and a generous seasoning of salt and pepper to create a savory egg creation.

4 SERVINGS

3 zucchini (8 ounces each), cut into ½-inch-thick rounds
1¼ teaspoons coarse salt
1 tablespoon extra virgin olive oil
4 green onions, thinly sliced
2 large cloves garlic, slivered
1 teaspoon fresh thyme leaves (or ½ teaspoon dried thyme leaves)

½ cup sliced green olives
1 teaspoon finely grated lemon peel
½ teaspoon coarse salt
½ teaspoon freshly ground pepper

PLACE the zucchini in a colander and sprinkle 1¼ teaspoons of salt on top; lightly blend. Allow the zucchini to sit for 30 minutes (this process removes any excess water). Rinse well. Pat dry with paper towels.

Heat a large skillet over medium-high heat for 1 minute. Add the olive oil and swirl the pan to coat the bottom evenly. Reduce the heat to medium-high. Add the zucchini, green onions, garlic, and thyme and cover the pan. Cook for 7 to 8 minutes or until the vegetables are tender, stirring occasionally. Add the olives, lemon peel, ½ teaspoon salt, and pepper and lightly blend.

EACH SERVING PROVIDES:
6g carbohydrates, 93 calories, 3g protein, 7g fat,
3g dietary fiber, 1566mg sodium, 0mg cholesterol

Zucchini Matchsticks

Who says you can't have your pasta and eat it, too! When you
sauté zucchini cut into matchsticks, you not only create a low-carb
vegetable that is delicious but also one that is very appealing to the
eye. To make a savory dish, add a bit of chopped garlic to the olive
oil before adding the zucchini.

4 SERVINGS

3 zucchini (8 ounces each),
   ends trimmed
1¼ teaspoons coarse salt
3 tablespoons extra virgin
   olive oil
1 teaspoon fresh lemon juice

½ teaspoon coarse salt
½ teaspoon freshly ground
   pepper
2 tablespoons chopped fresh
   parsley (optional)

CUT each zucchini in half horizontally. Cut each half vertically into
⅓- to ½-inch-thick slabs. Cut each slab into ⅓- to ½-inch-wide
matchsticks (it does not have to be exact). Place the zucchini in a colander and sprinkle 1¼ teaspoons of salt on top; lightly blend. Allow the
zucchini to sit for 30 minutes (this process removes any excess water).
Rinse well. Pat dry with paper towels.

Heat a large skillet over medium heat for 2 minutes. Add the olive
oil and swirl the pan to coat the bottom evenly. Add the zucchini
matchsticks and sauté for 3 to 4 minutes, stirring occasionally. Add
the lemon juice and season with ½ teaspoon salt and pepper; lightly
blend. Garnish each serving with chopped parsley, if desired.

EACH SERVING PROVIDES:
5g carbohydrates, 119 calories, 2g protein, 11g fat,
2g dietary fiber, 828mg sodium, 0mg cholesterol

Zucchini Pasta

Don't despair when you have a craving for pasta but are concerned about the carbohydrate content. You will be delighted with the taste, appearance, and texture of this easy-to-prepare all-vegetable pasta.

4 SERVINGS

4 medium zucchini, ends removed
1¼ teaspoons coarse salt

USING a vegetable peeler, slice the zucchini into long, thin strips, rotating it as you slice. (If the strips are too wide, cut them lengthwise into narrower strips.) Place the zucchini in a colander and sprinkle 1¼ teaspoons of salt on top; lightly blend. Allow the zucchini to sit for 30 minutes (this process removes any excess water). Rinse well.

Bring salted water to a rolling boil in a large saucepan. Add the zucchini and cook for 3 to 4 minutes or just until fork tender. Transfer the zucchini to a colander and drain well. Pat dry with paper towels.

EACH SERVING PROVIDES:
6g carbohydrates, 27 calories, 2g protein, 0g fat,
2g dietary fiber, 6mg sodium, 0mg cholesterol

Zucchini Soufflé

This soufflé is one of my favorite vegetable dishes to serve at a holiday meal. It can be assembled early in the day and baked just before serving.

6 SERVINGS

2 pounds (5 to 6 medium) zucchini, cut into ¼-inch-thick rounds
2 tablespoons butter
½ cup chopped yellow onion
1 clove garlic, chopped
4 eggs, well beaten

½ cup freshly grated Parmesan cheese
2 tablespoons 2 percent milk
½ teaspoon coarse salt
¼ teaspoon freshly ground pepper

PREHEAT the oven to 375 degrees F. Lightly coat a 2-quart soufflé or baking dish with a nonstick vegetable spray. Set aside.

Place the zucchini in a vegetable steamer filled with about 2 inches of boiling water. Steam for 15 minutes or until fork tender. Transfer the zucchini to a colander and drain well.

Meanwhile, melt the butter in a medium skillet over medium heat. Add the onion and garlic and cook, stirring occasionally, for 6 to 8 minutes or until soft.

Press down on the zucchini with the back of a spoon to extract as much water as possible. Place the zucchini in a medium bowl and add the onion mixture, eggs, cheese, milk, salt, and pepper and blend well. Spoon the zucchini mixture into the prepared baking dish and bake for 50 to 55 minutes or until set in the center. Serve immediately.

EACH SERVING PROVIDES:

7g carbohydrates, 145 calories, 9g protein, 10g fat,
2g dietary fiber, 394mg sodium, 142mg cholesterol

Zucchini and Swiss Cheese Soufflé

A friend gave me this recipe and insisted it was one of the best zucchini soufflés she had ever tasted. I have to admit that, after looking at the recipe, I was skeptical because of the simplicity of the ingredients. But don't be fooled like I was. This delicious vegetable dish will have you looking for any excuse to make it again and again.

6 SERVINGS

1½ pounds zucchini, cut into
    ¼-inch-thick rounds
½ cup whipping cream
3 ounces (¾ cup) shredded
    Swiss cheese

2 eggs, lightly beaten
½ teaspoon coarse salt
¼ teaspoon freshly ground
    pepper

PREHEAT oven to 350 degrees F. Lightly coat a 1½-quart baking dish with a nonstick vegetable spray. Set aside.

Bring salted water to a rolling boil in a large saucepan. Add the zucchini. Cover, and simmer for 10 to 12 minutes or until tender. Transfer the zucchini to a colander and drain well. Cool for at least 10 minutes.

Using the back of a large spoon, press down on the zucchini to remove as much liquid as possible. Combine the zucchini with the whipping cream, cheese, eggs, salt, and pepper in a medium bowl and blend well. Spoon the mixture into the prepared baking dish and bake for 45 to 50 minutes or until set in the center. Serve immediately.

EACH SERVING PROVIDES:

5g carbohydrates, 160 calories, 8g protein, 13g fat,
1g dietary fiber, 223mg sodium, 103mg cholesterol

chapter nine

DAZZLING
DESSERTS

✳ ✳ ✳ ✳ ✳ ✳ ✳ ✳ ✳

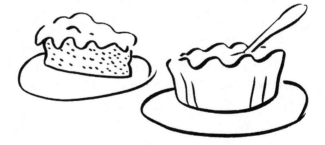

✳ ✳ ✳ ✳ ✳ ✳ ✳ ✳ ✳

DESSERTS

Muffins and Sweet Bread Temptations

Banana Cake

Banana, Chocolate Chip, and
    Walnut Muffins

Chocolate Chip and Almond
    Streusel Coffeecake

Pumpkin Gingerbread

Pumpkin and Walnut Bread

Pumpkin and Walnut Muffins

Yum Yum Coffeecake

Zucchini Bread

Bite-Size Indulgences

Chocolate Chip Meringue
    Cookies

Chocolate Chip and Pecan Bars

Chocolate Chip and Walnut
    Shortbread

Chocolate-Dipped Shortbread

Chocolate Peanut Butter Swirls

Chocolate Thumbprint
    Cookies

Chocolate Toffee Bars

Mandel Bread Cookies

Pecan Sandies

Pumpkin Bars

A Dessert for All Occasions

Baked Custard

Chocolate Coffee Pie

Crème Brûlée

Hazelnut Cake Roll

Italian Cake Roll

Lemon Chiffon Pie

Panna Cotta

Pecan Torte

Pumpkin Cake Roll

Pumpkin Cheesecake

Pumpkin Custard

The Ultimate Cheesecake

W HAT BETTER WAY TO describe a dessert than dazzling? With flavors that are brimming with sweetness and tastes and textures that are ravishingly rich
and creamy, it is no wonder that for many of us, dessert is
often the highlight of the meal. Unfortunately, as dazzling
as desserts can be, many of the ingredients that are usually re-
quired to create a confectionery masterpiece are not allowed
on a low-carbohydrate diet. Typical dessert ingredients such
as sugar, flour, many fruits, and some chocolates, just to
name a few, are so high in carbs, that even a small amount can
throw you out of ketosis and, what's worse, renew your cravings for more sweets and other forbidden high-carb foods.
But don't despair. There are ways to prepare decadent
desserts so "you can have your cake and eat it, too!"

In chapter 3, I discussed two sweeteners that are either
low in carbohydrates or metabolize differently than ordinary
sugar. Splenda, for example, is made from rearranged sugar
molecules, allowing it to pass through the body without being metabolized. It also does not affect the glucose level.
This means that although the carbohydrate count may be
similar to sugar, your body is not metabolizing it. By substituting stevia or Splenda for sugar, you can create equally delicious desserts without the worry.

I also have found that almond and high-gluten flour as
well as whey protein powder are excellent substitutes for all-
purpose flour in some recipes. By substituting chopped nuts
for the traditional graham cracker or butter cookie crusts that
are frequently the foundation of most cheesecakes or other
frozen desserts, you can still enjoy the rich and creamy filling without guilt. And what about chocolate, so rich in carbohydrates? It is no wonder we crave it. By simply reducing
the amount of chocolate called for in many recipes, you can

still derive its delectable and rich flavor but without an over-load of carbohydrates.

As I have mentioned in previous chapters, please don't hesitate to substitute low-fat or nonfat ingredients. In most instances, the flavor of the dessert will not be significantly compromised while the calorie count and fat grams can be greatly reduced. If you are seeking more ways to add soybean products to your diet, then try substituting tofu, soy milk, and soy yogurt for such dairy products as cream cheese, whole milk, or yogurt, as long as the carbohydrate count remains about the same.

This chapter was designed to satisfy your sweet tooth. I hope you will delight in the flavors of Panna Cotta, a richly creamy Italian dessert that can be served alone or topped with low-carbohydrate fruit. If chocolate is what you crave, then you will find Chocolate Toffee Bars a little taste of heaven. With 30 dazzling dessert recipes from which to choose, you will be sweetly rewarded for making a commitment to the low-carbohydrate way of dining.

MUFFINS AND SWEET
BREAD TEMPTATIONS

Although muffins and sweet breads are traditionally high in carbohydrate content, using novel low-carbohydrate ingredients will allow you to continue to enjoy these freshly baked pleasures without departing from your chosen diet plan.

Banana Cake

Banana cake is one of my all-time favorite comfort foods. My mother always saved her bananas that were turning brown so she could use them to make a delicious banana cake. For a very special treat, she would frost the cake with a rich chocolate icing—not exactly low-carb fare!

12 SERVINGS

1 cup vanilla whey protein powder
½ cup almond flour
2 teaspoons baking soda
¼ teaspoon coarse salt
6 tablespoons butter, at room temperature

2 large eggs
1¼ cups Splenda
1 teaspoon vanilla extract
¾ cup mashed ripe banana
½ cup sour cream

PREHEAT oven to 350 degrees F. Lightly coat an 8-inch square pan with a nonstick vegetable spray.

Combine the protein powder, almond flour, baking soda, and salt in a medium bowl and blend with a wire whisk. Set aside.

Place the butter in the mixing bowl of an electric mixer and beat on medium-high speed until light and fluffy. Add the eggs, one at a time, beating well after each addition and scraping down the sides of the bowl with a rubber spatula as necessary. Add the Splenda and beat for 3 minutes. Add the vanilla and blend. On medium-low speed, add the dry ingredients and beat until just blended, scraping down the sides of the bowl. Add the banana and sour cream and lightly blend. Spoon the batter into the prepared pan and smooth the top with a spatula. Bake for 20 to 25 minutes or until a cake tester inserted into the center of the cake comes out clean.

Remove the pan from the oven and place on a cooling rack. Cover with a piece of waxed paper and cool completely. When cool, remove the waxed paper and store the Banana Cake in an airtight container in the refrigerator.

ABOUT SPLENDA

Splenda is an excellent sugar replacement that can be used to create a variety of low-carbohydrate desserts. However, there are some important tips and techniques you should know when using this product, whether you are following the recipes in this chapter or adapting some of your favorites. Before I list these tips, you should be aware of some peculiarities of this product. I found that it is very important that the butter be at room temperature before beating it until light and fluffy. Once beaten, the eggs should be added, one at a time, before adding the Splenda. By following this technique, my sweet breads came out as tender as those made with ordinary sugar and flour.

Now, for the tips:

1. Use Splenda—cup for cup, or spoon for spoon—in place of sugar.
2. Incorporate Splenda into a recipe using the following three techniques:
   - Combine it thoroughly with the other dry ingredients
   - Dissolve it in liquid.
   - When a recipe does not call for eggs, cream it with butter or fat for at least three minutes to get enough air into the mixture.
3. Store baked goods made with Splenda in the refrigerator for lasting freshness.
4. Replace sugar with Splenda so your cakes will get done seven to ten minutes sooner, and cookies one to two minutes sooner.
5. When making a cake with Splenda, add ½ teaspoon baking soda for every cup of Splenda, or ½ cup nonfat dry milk. Add the baking soda with the dry ingredients.
6. When making cookies, bars, muffins, and quick breads, add ½ teaspoon baking soda for every 1 cup Splenda. The Splenda should be beaten with the butter, and the baking soda added to the dry ingredients.

Banana, Chocolate Chip, and Walnut Muffins

These tasty bite-size gems make a quick and easy breakfast or a welcomed treat nestled in a lunch box. If your taste leans toward banana and walnut muffins, simply omit the chocolate chips and add extra walnuts.

12 MUFFINS

¾ cup vanilla whey protein powder
¼ cup high-gluten flour
1½ teaspoons baking powder
¾ teaspoon baking soda
½ teaspoon ground cinnamon
½ teaspoon coarse salt
½ cup (1 stick) butter, melted and cooled slightly

1 cup Splenda
1 cup mashed ripe banana
⅓ cup milk
1 large egg
¾ cup chopped walnuts
½ cup Zero-Carb chocolate chips*

PREHEAT oven to 350 degrees F. Line muffin tins with paper cupcake holders. Set aside.

Combine the protein powder, gluten flour, baking powder, baking soda, cinnamon, and salt in a medium bowl and blend with a wire whisk.

Combine the butter and Splenda in another medium bowl and beat with a whisk for 2 minutes. Add the banana, milk, and egg and blend well. Add the dry ingredients and mix with a fork until just blended. Fold in the walnuts and chocolate chips. Spoon the batter into the prepared muffin tin, two-thirds full. Bake for 12 to 15 minutes or until firm to the touch.

*Zero-Carb chocolate chips can be purchased on the Web (www.lowcarboutfitters.com).

Remove the muffin tin from the oven and place it on a cooling rack. When cool, store the Banana, Chocolate Chip, and Walnut Muffins in an airtight container in the refrigerator.

11g carbohydrates, 234 calories, 9g protein, 17g fat,
1g dietary fiber, 241mg sodium, 48mg cholesterol

Chocolate Chip and Almond Streusel Coffeecake

A low-carbohydrate dessert made with chocolate chips sounds too good to be true. Thanks to Zero-Carb chocolate chips, dieting has never been more rewarding. Each little morsel adds a divine flavor to an already scrumptious delight.

12 SERVINGS

Almond Streusel Topping
¼ cup Splenda
¼ cup almond flour
2 tablespoons butter, well
   chilled and cut into 8 pieces
6 tablespoons sliced almonds
¼ cup Zero-Carb chocolate
   chips*

Coffeecake
¾ cup vanilla whey protein
   powder
¼ cup almond flour
¾ teaspoon baking soda
½ teaspoon baking powder
¼ teaspoon coarse salt
5 tablespoons butter, at room
   temperature
2 large eggs
¾ cup Splenda
¼ cup milk
½ teaspoon almond extract
¾ cup Zero-Carb chocolate
   chips

PREHEAT oven to 350 degrees F. Lightly coat a 9-inch round cake pan with a nonstick vegetable spray and dust with almond flour. Set aside.

To make the almond streusel, combine ¼ cup Splenda and almond flour in a medium bowl and blend. Using a pastry blender, cut in the butter until the mixture resembles coarse meal. Fold in the almonds and ¼ cup chocolate chips. Set aside.

*Zero-Carb chocolate chips can be purchased on the Web (www.lowcarboutfitters.com).

To make the coffeecake, combine the protein powder, almond flour, baking soda, baking powder, and salt in a medium bowl and blend with a wire whisk.

Place the butter in the mixing bowl of an electric mixer and beat on medium-high speed until light and fluffy. Add the eggs, one at a time, beating well after each addition and scraping down the sides of the bowl with a rubber spatula as necessary. Add ¾ cup Splenda and beat for 3 minutes. Add the milk and almond extract and blend. On medium-low speed, add the dry ingredients and beat until just blended. Fold in the chocolate chips. Spoon the batter into the prepared pan and sprinkle the Almond Streusel Topping over the top. Bake for 20 minutes or until a cake tester inserted into the center of the cake comes out clean.

Remove the pan from the oven and place it on a cooling rack. When cool, store the coffeecake in an airtight container in the refrigerator.

VARIATION: The coffeecake can be topped with a chocolate glaze by combining ¼ cup Zero-Carb chocolate chips, ½ tablespoon butter, and ½ teaspoon milk in a small saucepan, covered, over low heat. Cook until the chocolate is soft enough to blend. Remove the saucepan from the heat and blend the mixture until smooth. Drizzle the glaze over the cooled coffeecake.

EACH SERVING PROVIDES:
5g carbohydrates, 256 calories, 10g protein, 20g fat,
1g dietary fiber, 166mg sodium, 63mg cholesterol

Pumpkin Gingerbread

If you love pumpkin and adore gingerbread then this winning combination is destined to become one of your favorite low-carb sweets. The bread is bursting with spices and flavors that linger long after the last bite.

16 SERVINGS

1¼ cups vanilla whey protein powder

¾ cup almond flour

2 teaspoons ground ginger

1 teaspoon baking soda

½ teaspoon ground cinnamon

½ teaspoon ground nutmeg

½ teaspoon coarse salt

¼ teaspoon ground cloves

¼ teaspoon dry mustard

¼ teaspoon baking powder

6 tablespoons butter, at room temperature

2 large eggs

1½ cups Splenda

2 tablespoons coffee*

¾ cup solid-packed pumpkin

1 cup chopped walnuts or pecans (optional)

PREHEAT oven to 350 degrees F. Lightly coat a 9 × 5-inch loaf pan with a nonstick vegetable spray and dust with almond flour. Set aside.

Combine the protein powder, almond flour, ginger, baking soda, cinnamon, nutmeg, salt, cloves, mustard, and baking powder in a medium bowl and blend with a wire whisk.

Place the butter in the mixing bowl of an electric mixer and beat on medium-high speed until light and fluffy. Add the eggs, one at a time, beating well after each addition and scraping down the sides of the bowl with a rubber spatula as necessary. Add the Splenda and beat for 3 minutes. On medium-low speed, alternately add the dry ingredients and coffee, beginning and ending with the dry ingredients. Beat

*Combine 2 tablespoons hot water with ½ teaspoon instant powdered coffee.

until just blended, scraping down the sides of the bowl. Add the pumpkin and optional nuts and lightly blend. Spoon the batter into the prepared pan and smooth the top with a spatula. Bake for 40 to 45 minutes or until a cake tester inserted into the center of the bread comes out clean. Remove the pan from the oven and place on a cooling rack. Cover with a piece of waxed paper and cool for 10 minutes. Remove the waxed paper. Cover the pan with a rack and invert it. Remove the pan, and turn the bread over again. Re-cover with waxed paper and cool completely. When cool, remove the waxed paper and store the gingerbread in an airtight container in the refrigerator.

EACH SERVING PROVIDES:

6g carbohydrates, 129 calories, 8g protein, 9g fat,
1g dietary fiber, 171mg sodium, 49mg cholesterol

Pumpkin and Walnut Bread

When you live in the Midwest, where winters can be frightfully cold, pumpkin bread gets high ratings as one of the all-time favorite comfort foods. But cold weather is not a prerequisite for indulging in this delicious and satisfying bread; it is a treat for all seasons.

12 TO 16 SERVINGS

1 cup vanilla whey protein
   powder
½ cup almond flour
1½ teaspoons baking soda
¾ teaspoon ground cinnamon
½ teaspoon baking powder
½ teaspoon coarse salt
½ teaspoon ground allspice

¼ teaspoon ground nutmeg
1¼ cups Splenda
1 cup solid-packed pumpkin
⅓ cup canola oil
2 large eggs
¼ cup warm water
½ cup (or more) chopped
   walnuts

PREHEAT oven to 350 degrees F. Lightly coat a 9 × 5-inch loaf pan with a nonstick vegetable spray. Set aside.

Combine the protein powder, almond flour, baking soda, cinnamon, baking powder, salt, allspice, and nutmeg in a medium bowl and blend with a wire whisk.

Combine the Splenda, pumpkin, canola oil, and eggs in a large bowl and whisk for 2 minutes. Gradually add the dry ingredients and blend well, scraping down the sides of the bowl with a rubber spatula as necessary. Add the water, 2 to 3 tablespoons at a time, and blend after each addition. Fold in the walnuts. Spoon the batter into the prepared pan and smooth the top with a spatula. Bake for 45 to 50 minutes or until a cake tester inserted into the center of the bread comes out clean.

Remove the pan from the oven and place on a cooling rack. Cover with a piece of waxed paper and cool for 10 minutes. Remove the waxed paper. Cover the pan with a rack and invert it. Remove the pan, and turn the bread over again. Re-cover with waxed paper and cool completely. When cool, remove the waxed paper and store the bread in an airtight container in the refrigerator.

EACH SERVING PROVIDES:

8g carbohydrates, 180 calories, 9g protein, 13g fat,
2g dietary fiber, 286mg sodium, 47mg cholesterol

Pumpkin and Walnut Muffins

Don't wait for Halloween to make these sensationally spicy muffins. Enjoy them year-round for breakfast, as a snack, or with a hearty dinner.

8 MUFFINS

½ cup vanilla whey protein powder

¼ cup almond flour

½ teaspoon baking soda

¼ teaspoon baking powder

1 teaspoon ground cinnamon

½ teaspoon ground ginger

¼ teaspoon ground cloves

¼ teaspoon ground nutmeg

⅛ teaspoon ground allspice

⅛ teaspoon coarse salt

6 tablespoons butter, melted and cooled slightly

⅔ cup Splenda

½ cup solid-packed pumpkin

1 large egg

1 teaspoon vanilla extract

½ cup chopped walnuts

PREHEAT oven to 350 degrees F. Line muffin tins with paper cupcake holders. Set aside.

Combine the protein powder, almond flour, baking soda, baking powder, cinnamon, ginger, cloves, nutmeg, allspice, and salt in a medium bowl and blend with a wire whisk.

Combine the butter and Splenda in another medium bowl and whisk for 2 minutes. Add the pumpkin, egg, and vanilla and blend well. Add the dry ingredients and mix with a fork until just blended. Fold in the walnuts. Spoon the batter into the prepared muffin tin, two-thirds full. Bake for 15 minutes or until firm to the touch.

Remove the muffin tin from the oven and place it on a cooling rack. Cool completely. Store the muffins in an airtight container in the refrigerator.

EACH SERVING PROVIDES:
7g carbohydrates, 198 calories, 8g protein, 16g fat,
1g dietary fiber, 147mg sodium, 59mg cholesterol

Yum Yum Coffeecake

This is one of my favorite recipes for coffeecake. It is moist and deliciously rich in flavor. If you are not losing weight as quickly as desired, you can substitute pureed nonfat cottage cheese for the sour cream. The cake remains flavorful and is a welcoming treat for low-carb dieters.

20 SERVINGS

Walnut Filling
¾ cup coarsely chopped walnuts
6 tablespoons Splenda
1 teaspoon ground cinnamon

Coffeecake
1¼ cups vanilla whey protein
   powder
¾ cup almond flour
1½ teaspoons baking soda

1 teaspoon baking powder
¼ teaspoon coarse salt
6 tablespoons butter, at room
   temperature
2 large eggs
1 cup Splenda
1 teaspoon vanilla extract
1 cup sour cream (or pureed
   nonfat cottage cheese)

PREHEAT oven to 350 degrees F. Lightly coat a 9-inch baking pan with a nonstick vegetable spray. Set aside.

To make the Walnut Filling, combine all the ingredients and blend well. Set aside.

To make the coffeecake, combine the protein powder, almond flour, baking soda, baking powder, and salt in a medium bowl and blend with a wire whisk.

Place the butter in the mixing bowl of an electric mixer and beat on medium-high speed until light and fluffy. Add the eggs, one at a time, beating well after each addition and scraping down the sides of the bowl with a rubber spatula as necessary. Add 1 cup Splenda and

(continues)

beat for 3 minutes. Add the vanilla and blend. On medium-low speed, alternately add the dry ingredients and sour cream, beginning and ending with the dry ingredients. Beat until just blended, scraping down the sides of the bowl.

Spread one-half of the batter in the prepared pan. Sprinkle half of the Walnut Filling over the batter. Drop the remaining batter by spoonfuls over the Walnut Filling. Using a metal spatula, spread the batter in an even layer. Sprinkle the remaining Walnut Filling over the batter. Bake for 25 minutes or until a cake tester inserted into the center of the cake comes out clean.

Remove the pan from the oven and place on a cooling rack. Cool completely. Store the coffeecake in an airtight container in the refrigerator.

EACH SERVING PROVIDES:

5g carbohydrates, 151 calories, 7g protein, 11g fat,
1g dietary fiber, 168mg sodium, 49mg cholesterol

Zucchini Bread

You will be amazed that zucchini could create such a deliciously moist bread. Laced with cinnamon and walnuts, this bread has just enough sweetness to serve with morning coffee or to satisfy a latent sweet tooth.

12 TO 16 SERVINGS

1¼ cups vanilla whey protein powder

¾ cup almond flour

2½ teaspoons ground cinnamon

1 teaspoon baking soda

½ teaspoon baking powder

⅛ teaspoon coarse salt

¾ pound zucchini, ends trimmed

1¼ cups Splenda

¾ cup canola oil

2 large eggs

¾ teaspoon vanilla extract

½ cup (or more) chopped walnuts

PREHEAT oven to 350 degrees F. Lightly coat a 9 × 5-inch loaf pan with a nonstick vegetable spray. Set aside.

Combine the protein powder, almond flour, cinnamon, baking soda, baking powder, and salt in a medium bowl and blend with a wire whisk.

Place the zucchini in the work bowl of a food processor fitted with a metal blade (or in a blender) and process until finely chopped.

Combine the Splenda, canola oil, eggs, and vanilla in the mixing bowl of an electric mixer and beat on medium-high speed for 2 minutes. On medium-low speed, add the dry ingredients and blend well, scraping down the sides of the bowl with a rubber spatula as necessary. Add the zucchini and any liquid remaining in the work bowl and mix with a wooden spoon or spatula until blended (the mixture will be thick). Fold in the walnuts. Spoon the batter into the prepared pan and smooth the top with a spatula. Bake for 1 hour or until a cake tester inserted into the center of the bread comes out clean.

(continues)

Remove the pan from the oven and place on a cooling rack. Cover with a piece of waxed paper and cool for 10 minutes. Remove the waxed paper. Cover the pan with a rack and invert it. Remove the pan, and turn the bread over again. Re-cover with waxed paper and cool completely. When cool, remove the waxed paper and store the bread in an airtight container in the refrigerator.

EACH SERVING PROVIDES:

8g carbohydrates, 269 calories, 11g protein, 22g fat,
2g dietary fiber, 178mg sodium, 50mg cholesterol

BITE-SIZE INDULGENCES

Surprise! Cookies are not necessarily off-limits for low-carbohydrate dining. Baking with novel low-carb ingredients will allow you to enjoy these previously sinful morsels without guilt.

Chocolate Chip Meringue Cookies

After placing these cookies in a preheated oven, the heat is turned off and you "forget" about the cookies being there for the next 8 hours. It is hard to believe this technique could produce such sweet little gems.

36 COOKIES

2 large egg whites, at room
   temperature
⅛ teaspoon coarse salt
¾ cup Splenda

1 teaspoon vanilla extract
¾ cup Zero-Carb chocolate
   chips*

PREHEAT oven to 350 degrees F. Line a baking sheet with a piece of aluminum foil. Set aside.

Place the egg whites in the mixing bowl of an electric mixer and beat on medium-high speed until foamy. Add the salt and blend. Gradually add the Splenda and beat until stiff. Fold in the vanilla and chocolate chips. Drop rounded teaspoonfuls of egg-white mixture onto the prepared baking sheet, 2 inches apart. Place the baking sheet in the oven. Turn off the oven heat. Leave the cookies in the oven for 8 hours or overnight, but be certain not to open the oven door during this time.

EACH SERVING PROVIDES:

1g carbohydrates, 28 calories, 1g protein, 2g fat,
0g dietary fiber, 10mg sodium, 0mg cholesterol

*Zero-Carb chocolate chips can be purchased on the Web (www.lowcarboutfitters.com).

Chocolate Chip and Pecan Bars

These low-carbohydrate bars are as delicious as eating a chocolate chip cookie. Thanks to the Zero-Carb chocolate chips, you can actually have your bar and eat it, too.

24 BARS

1 cup high-gluten flour
¼ cup vanilla whey protein
    powder
½ teaspoon baking soda
¼ teaspoon coarse salt
½ cup (1 stick) butter, at room
    temperature
¾ cup Splenda

1 teaspoon powdered white
    stevia
1 large egg
1 teaspoon vanilla extract
1 cup finely chopped pecans
1 cup Zero-Carb chocolate
    chips*

PREHEAT oven to 375 degrees F. Lightly coat a 9-inch baking pan with a nonstick vegetable spray. Set aside.

Combine the gluten flour, protein powder, baking soda, and salt in a medium bowl and blend with a wire whisk.

Place the butter, Splenda, and stevia in the mixing bowl of an electric mixer and beat on medium-high speed for 3 minutes, scraping down the sides of the bowl with a rubber spatula as necessary. Add the egg and vanilla and beat for 1 minute. Add the pecans and blend well. On medium-low speed, add the dry ingredients and mix until the dough begins to stick together (it will not be a smooth dough but will hold together when pressed in the pan). Add the chocolate chips and blend well. Press the dough evenly into the prepared pan. Bake for 17 to 18 minutes or until golden brown.

(continues)

*Zero-Carb chocolate chips can be purchased on the Web (www.lowcarboutfitters.com).

Remove the pan from the oven and place on a cooling rack. Cool for 15 minutes. Cut into bars and cool completely. Store the bars in an airtight container in the refrigerator.

EACH SERVING PROVIDES:

6g carbohydrates, 144 calories, 3g protein, 11g fat,
0g dietary fiber, 52mg sodium, 21mg cholesterol

Chocolate Chip and Walnut Shortbread

These are positively the best chocolate chip bars you will have ever tasted. Loaded with Zero-Carb chocolate chips, the chocoholic in you will definitely be satisfied.

18 TO 24 BARS

1 cup high-gluten flour
¾ cup vanilla whey protein
    powder
½ teaspoon baking soda
1 stick plus 2 tablespoons
    butter, at room temperature

½ cup Splenda
½ teaspoon powdered white
    stevia
1 cup finely chopped walnuts
1 cup Zero-Carb chocolate
    chips*

PREHEAT oven to 350 degrees F. Lightly coat an 8-inch baking pan with a nonstick vegetable spray. Set aside.

Combine the gluten flour, protein powder, and baking soda in a medium bowl and blend with a wire whisk.

Place the butter, Splenda, and stevia in the mixing bowl of an electric mixer and beat on medium-high speed for 3 minutes, scraping down the sides of the bowl with a rubber spatula as necessary. Add the walnuts and blend well. On medium-low speed, add the dry ingredients and mix until the dough begins to stick together (it will not be a smooth dough but will hold together when pressed in the pan). Add the chocolate chips and blend well. Press the dough into the prepared pan. Bake for 45 to 50 minutes or until golden brown.

(continues)

*Zero-Carb chocolate chips can be purchased on the Web (www.lowcarboutfitters.com).

Remove the pan from the oven and place on a cooling rack. Cool for 15 minutes. Cut into bars and cool completely. Store the shortbread in an airtight container in the refrigerator.

EACH SERVING PROVIDES:

7g carbohydrates, 229 calories, 7g protein, 18g fat,
0g dietary fiber, 45mg sodium, 30mg cholesterol

Chocolate-Dipped Shortbread

I love to make these cookies when I am serving a platter arranged with an assortment of sweets. These exceptionally rich sweet indulgences have real eye appeal as well as being delicious.

42 TO 48 COOKIES

½ cup (or more) finely ground walnuts or pecans

Shortbread
1½ cups high-gluten flour
½ cup vanilla whey protein powder
½ teaspoon baking soda
1 cup (2 sticks) butter, at room temperature

½ cup Splenda
1 teaspoon powdered white stevia
1 teaspoon vanilla extract

Chocolate Topping
5 to 6 ounces Darrell Lea Sugar Free Milk Chocolate or favorite sugar-free chocolate, coarsely chopped*

Preheat oven to 350 degrees F. Line a baking sheet with a piece of parchment paper. Line another baking sheet with a piece of waxed paper. Place the walnuts in a small dish. Set aside.

Combine the gluten flour, protein powder, and baking soda in a medium bowl and blend with a wire whisk.

Place the butter, Splenda, and stevia in the mixing bowl of an electric mixer and beat on medium-high speed for 3 minutes, scraping down the sides of the bowl as necessary. Add the vanilla and blend well. On medium-low speed, add the dry ingredients and beat until the dough begins to stick together (it will not be a smooth dough). Using your hands, work the dough just until it holds together. Roll the dough

(continues)

*Darrell Lea Sugar Free Milk Chocolate can be purchased online at: www.lowcarb outfitters.com.

into 2-inch logs and place them on the parchment-lined baking sheet, 1 inch apart. Bake for 8 to 10 minutes or just until the edges begin to brown.

Remove the baking sheet from the oven and place it on a cooling rack. Cool completely.

For the Chocolate Topping, melt the chocolate in a small heavy saucepan (or in the microwave), covered, over very low heat, stirring occasionally.

When the chocolate has melted, dip one end of each cookie in it and then roll the dipped end in the walnuts. Place the cookies on the waxed paper–lined cookie sheet and refrigerate until the chocolate has set. Store the shortbread in an airtight container in the refrigerator.

EACH SERVING PROVIDES:

4g carbohydrates, 84 calories, 2g protein, 7g fat,

0g dietary fiber, 22mg sodium, 14mg cholesterol

Chocolate Peanut Butter Swirls

Who doesn't adore the classic combination of chocolate and peanut butter? These cookies are the absolute ultimate in taste and appearance for this wonderful duet.

24 COOKIES

Chocolate Dough
6 tablespoons butter, at room temperature
½ cup Splenda
½ teaspoon powdered white stevia
1 large egg
1 teaspoon vanilla extract
1½ ounces unsweetened chocolate, melted
1 cup almond flour

¼ teaspoon baking soda
¼ teaspoon coarse salt

Peanut Butter Dough
½ cup Splenda
¼ cup creamy natural peanut butter
2 tablespoons butter, at room temperature
2 tablespoons almond flour

PREHEAT oven to 350 degrees F. Line a baking sheet with a piece of parchment paper. Set aside.

To make the Chocolate Dough, put the butter in the mixing bowl of an electric mixer and beat on medium-high speed until creamy. Add the Splenda and stevia and beat for 3 minutes. Add the egg and vanilla and blend. Add the melted chocolate and blend well, scraping down the sides of the bowl with a rubber spatula as necessary. On medium-low speed, gradually add 1 cup almond flour, baking soda, and salt and beat until smooth, scraping down the sides of the bowl.

To make the Peanut Butter Dough, put all the ingredients in a clean mixing bowl and beat until smooth.

To make the cookies, divide the Chocolate Dough in half. Place each half in a separate bowl. Set one bowl aside.

(continues)

Drop rounded teaspoonfuls of Chocolate Dough onto the prepared baking sheet, 2 inches apart. Drop a scant teaspoonful of Peanut Butter Dough on top of each cookie and then top each cookie with a teaspoonful of Chocolate Dough remaining in the bowl that was set aside. Using the tines of a fork dipped in Splenda, flatten each cookie. Bake for 15 minutes.

Remove the baking sheet from the oven and place it on a cooling rack. Cool completely. Store the Chocolate Peanut Butter Swirl cookies in an airtight container in the refrigerator.

EACH SERVING PROVIDES:
3g carbohydrates, 102 calories, 2g protein, 9g fat,
1g dietary fiber, 37mg sodium, 19mg cholesterol

Chocolate Thumbprint Cookies

One taste of these richly chocolate-flavored, bite-size gems will confirm your commitment to the low-carb way of eating. Tuck a couple in your lunch box or savor one during an afternoon coffee break—you deserve to be sweetly rewarded. This recipe can be doubled easily.

24 COOKIES

Chocolate Cookies
½ cup almond flour
½ cup high-gluten flour
¼ teaspoon baking soda
¼ teaspoon coarse salt
3 tablespoons Dutch process
  cocoa (unsweetened
  alkalized)
1 tablespoon canola oil
6 tablespoons butter, at room
  temperature

½ cup Splenda
1 large egg yolk
1 teaspoon vanilla extract

Chocolate Topping
8 ounces Darrell Lea Sugar
  Free Milk Chocolate or favorite sugar-free chocolate,
  coarsely chopped*
24 small toasted pecan halves**

PREHEAT oven to 350 degrees F. Line a baking sheet with a piece of parchment paper. Set aside.

To make the Chocolate Cookies, combine the almond flour, gluten flour, baking soda, and salt in a medium bowl and blend with a wire whisk.

Combine the cocoa and canola oil in a small bowl and blend well.

(continues)

---

*Darrell Lea Sugar Free Milk Chocolate can be purchased online at: www.lowcarb outfitters.com.

**To toast the pecans: Preheat the oven to 350 degrees F, place the nuts in a shallow pan, and bake for 5 minutes.

Place the butter in the mixing bowl of an electric mixer and beat on medium speed until creamy. Add the Splenda and beat for 3 minutes. Add the egg yolk and blend well, scraping down the sides of the bowl with a rubber spatula as necessary. Add the chocolate mixture and the vanilla and blend well. On medium-low speed, gradually add the dry ingredients and beat until the dough begins to stick together (it will not be a smooth dough). Using your hands, work the dough just until it holds together.

Pinch off small pieces of dough and roll them between the palm of your hands to form 1-inch balls. Place the balls on the prepared baking sheet, 1 inch apart. Using your thumb, make an indentation in the center of each ball. Bake for 10 minutes.

Remove the pan from the oven and place on a cooling rack. Cool completely.

To make the Chocolate Topping, place the chocolate in a small saucepan. Cover, and cook over low heat until melted. Blend until smooth. (The chocolate also can be placed in a medium dish, covered with plastic wrap, and set on the hot plate of a coffee maker. Turn the coffee maker on and the chocolate will slowly melt. Stir occasionally.)

Spoon some of the melted chocolate in the indentation of each cookie. Place a pecan in the center of the chocolate. Arrange the cookies on a baking sheet and refrigerate until firm. Once firm, transfer the cookies to an airtight container and store in the refrigerator.

EACH SERVING PROVIDES:
4g carbohydrates, 114 calories, 2g protein, 10g fat,
1g dietary fiber, 47mg sodium, 17mg cholesterol

Chocolate Toffee Bars

My mother used to make these chocolate toffee bars, and I absolutely adored them. To keep the carbohydrates at a minimum, I made some major substitutions for the high-carb ingredients called for in the recipe, and the bars are still irresistibly delicious.

24 BARS

1½ cups high-gluten flour
½ cup vanilla whey protein
  powder
½ teaspoon baking soda
¼ teaspoon coarse salt
15 tablespoons (1 stick plus 7
  tablespoons) butter, at room
  temperature
¾ cup Splenda
1 teaspoon powdered white
  stevia

1 large egg yolk
1 teaspoon vanilla extract
6 ounces Darrell Lea Sugar
  Free Milk Chocolate or
  favorite sugar-free chocolate,
  coarsely chopped*
½ cup chopped walnuts or
  pecans

PREHEAT oven to 375 degrees F. Lightly coat a rimmed baking sheet with a nonstick vegetable spray. Set aside.

Combine the gluten flour, protein powder, baking soda, and salt in a medium bowl and blend with a wire whisk.

Place the butter, Splenda, and stevia in the mixing bowl of an electric mixer and beat on medium-high speed for 3 minutes, scraping down the sides of the bowl as necessary. Add the egg yolk and vanilla and blend well. On medium-low speed, add the dry ingredients and beat until the dough begins to stick together (it will not be a smooth

(continues)

*Darrell Lea Sugar Free Milk Chocolate can be purchased online at: www.lowcarb outfitters.com.

dough but will hold together when pressed in the pan). Press the dough in the prepared pan to make an even layer that completely covers the bottom of the pan. Bake for 12 to 15 minutes or until golden brown.

Remove the pan from the oven and place it on a cooling rack. Immediately distribute the chocolate pieces all over the bars and allow them to sit for at least 2 minutes. Using a metal spatula, spread the melted chocolate to completely cover the bars. Sprinkle chopped nuts over the chocolate. Cut into bars while still warm. When cool, store the bars in an airtight container in the refrigerator.

EACH SERVING PROVIDES:
7g carbohydrates, 152 calories, 4g protein, 12g fat,
0g dietary fiber, 62mg sodium, 31mg cholesterol

Mandel Bread Cookies

These cookies are similar in taste and texture to biscotti. They are crisp and crunchy and bursting with the flavor of almonds.

48 COOKIES

1½ cups almond flour
1 cup vanilla whey protein
   powder
1½ teaspoons baking powder
½ teaspoon baking soda
½ teaspoon coarse salt
½ cup (1 stick) butter, at room
   temperature

¾ cup Splenda
1 teaspoon powdered white
   stevia
3 large eggs
1¼ cups finely chopped
   blanched almonds

PREHEAT oven to 350 degrees F. Line a baking sheet with a piece of parchment paper. Set aside.

Combine the almond flour, protein powder, baking powder, baking soda, and salt in a medium bowl and blend with a wire whisk.

Place the butter, Splenda, and stevia in the mixing bowl of an electric mixer and beat on medium-high speed for 3 minutes, scraping down the sides of the bowl with a rubber spatula as necessary. Add the eggs, one at a time, scraping down the sides of the bowl. On medium-low speed, add the dry ingredients and blend well. Add the almonds and lightly blend.

Divide the dough into two sections. Form two 12-inch logs on the prepared baking sheet, placing them 4 inches apart (the cookies will spread during the baking process). Bake for 20 minutes.

Remove the pan from the oven and place on a cooling rack. Cool for 10 minutes.

(continues)

Reduce oven temperature to 325 degrees F. Using a serrated knife, cut each log into ½-inch slices. Lay each slice flat on the baking sheet. Bake for 10 to 12 minutes or until crisp, turning the cookies over halfway through the cooking time.

Remove the pan from the oven and place it on a cooling rack. Cool completely. Store the cookies in an airtight container in the refrigerator.

EACH SERVING PROVIDES:

2g carbohydrates, 76 calories, 3g protein, 6g fat,
1g dietary fiber, 57mg sodium, 21mg cholesterol

Pecan Sandies

Everyone seems to have a favorite recipe for pecan sandies—and for good reason. These cookies are decadently sweet and almost melt in your mouth. Their only downfall is that they are laden with carbohydrates. The good news is that by making substitutions for a few of the traditional high-carb ingredients, you can now enjoy these sensational cookies while following a low-carb regimen.

36 COOKIES

1 cup high-gluten flour
$\frac{2}{3}$ cup vanilla whey protein
  powder
$\frac{2}{3}$ cup finely chopped pecans
$\frac{1}{8}$ teaspoon coarse salt
1 cup (2 sticks) butter, at room
  temperature

$\frac{1}{3}$ cup Splenda
1 teaspoon powdered white
  stevia
1 teaspoon vanilla extract

PREHEAT oven to 350 degrees F. Line a baking sheet with a piece of parchment paper. Set aside.

Combine the gluten flour, protein powder, pecans, and salt in a medium bowl and blend with a wire whisk.

Place the butter, Splenda, and stevia in the mixing bowl of an electric mixer and beat on medium-high speed for 3 minutes, scraping down the sides of the bowl with a rubber spatula as necessary. Add the vanilla and blend. On medium-low speed, add the dry ingredients and mix until the dough begins to stick together (it will not be a smooth dough). Using your hands, work the dough just until it holds together. Roll the dough into $\frac{3}{4}$- to 1-inch balls and place them on the prepared baking sheet, 1 inch apart. Slightly flatten each cookie with your fingertips. Bake for 15 minutes or just until the edges begin to brown.

(continues)

Remove the baking sheet from the oven and place it on a cooling rack. Cool completely. Store the Pecan Sandies in an airtight container in the refrigerator.

EACH SERVING PROVIDES:

3g carbohydrates, 80 calories, 2g protein, 7g fat,

0g dietary fiber, 11mg sodium, 16mg cholesterol

Pumpkin Bars

These pumpkin bars have a wonderful cakelike consistency. Iced with a traditional cream cheese frosting (sans powdered sugar), you get double the taste treat.

18 BARS

Pumpkin Bars
½ cup high-gluten flour
½ cup vanilla whey protein
    powder
1 teaspoon ground cinnamon
1 teaspoon baking powder
½ teaspoon baking soda
⅛ teaspoon coarse salt
¾ cup solid-packed pumpkin
1 cup Splenda
⅓ cup canola oil
2 large eggs

Cream Cheese Frosting
½ cup Splenda
4 tablespoons cream cheese, at
    room temperature
2 tablespoons butter, at room
    temperature
2 tablespoons whipping cream
½ teaspoon vanilla extract
    (optional)

PREHEAT oven to 350 degrees F. Lightly coat an 8-inch square pan with a nonstick vegetable spray. Set aside.

To make the Pumpkin Bars, combine the gluten flour, protein powder, cinnamon, baking powder, baking soda, and salt in a medium bowl and blend with a wire whisk.

Combine the pumpkin, 1 cup Splenda, canola oil, and eggs in a large mixing bowl and mix with a fork until well blended. Add the dry ingredients and blend well. Spoon the batter into the prepared pan and smooth the top with a spatula. Bake for 18 minutes or until a cake tester inserted in the center of the cake comes out clean.

Remove the pan from the oven and place on a cooling rack. Cool completely.

(continues)

To make the Cream Cheese Frosting, combine ½ cup Splenda, cream cheese, and butter in a mixing bowl and beat with a hand-held beater until well blended. Add the whipping cream and optional vanilla and beat until well blended.

Spread the Cream Cheese Frosting over the cooled Pumpkin Bars. Place the Pumpkin Bars in the refrigerator. When the Cream Cheese Frosting has set, cover the pan with a piece of aluminum foil.

EACH SERVING PROVIDES:

6g carbohydrates, 106 calories, 3g protein, 8g fat,
0g dietary fiber, 100mg sodium, 37mg cholesterol

Dazzling Desserts
••••

A DESSERT FOR ALL OCCASIONS

When you crave a satisfying dessert or want to please your guests with an impressive after-meal offering, don't overlook the surprisingly rich and sweet temptations described in this section. You will be amazed that these seductively rich creations are "legal" on a low-carbohydrate diet.

Baked Custard

Vanilla-scented custard is one of the ultimate comfort foods. With every spoonful of this rich and creamy reward, you will be happy you chose the low-carb way of dining.

8 TO 10 SERVINGS

½ cup Splenda
3 large eggs
2 large egg yolks
¼ teaspoon powdered white
   stevia

3 cups milk
1 teaspoon vanilla extract
¼ teaspoon ground nutmeg
   or ginger

PREHEAT oven to 350 degrees F. Combine the Splenda, eggs, egg yolks, and stevia in a medium bowl and beat for 2 minutes with a wire whisk until thick.

Meanwhile, bring the milk to a boil in a heavy medium saucepan over medium heat. Gradually add the hot milk to the egg mixture, whisking constantly. Add the vanilla and blend well.

Pour the mixture into a 1-quart soufflé dish and sprinkle nutmeg all over. Place the dish in a larger pan and put in the oven. Pour enough hot water into the pan to come halfway up the sides of the dish. Bake for 40 minutes or until the custard is firm.

Remove the dish from the oven and place on a cooling rack. When cool, refrigerate the custard for several hours.

EACH SERVING PROVIDES:
6g carbohydrates, 107 calories, 6g protein, 6g fat,
0g dietary fiber, 72mg sodium, 145mg cholesterol

Chocolate Coffee Pie

You only need a few bites of this heavenly dessert to appreciate its complexity of flavors. This sensational pie is composed of an intensely rich mocha filling nestled in a flaky crust and topped with coffee-flavored whipped cream—need I say more?

12 SERVINGS

Crust
1 cup high-gluten flour
⅓ cup almond flour
1½ tablespoons Splenda
½ teaspoon coarse salt
2 tablespoons milk
½ cup canola oil

Chocolate Coffee Filling
½ cup (1 stick) butter, at room temperature
¾ cup Splenda
1 square (1 ounce) unsweetened chocolate (or 2 ounces Darrell Lea Sugar Free Milk Chocolate), melted*

1 teaspoon instant powdered coffee
2 large eggs

Coffee Topping
1 cup whipping cream
½ tablespoon instant powdered coffee
¼ cup Splenda

PREHEAT oven to 400 degrees F.
  To make the crust, combine the gluten flour, almond flour, 1½ tablespoons Splenda, and salt in a large bowl and blend with a fork. Add the milk and canola oil and mix until well blended. Press the dough into a 9-inch pie pan. Bake for 10 minutes.

(continues)

*Darrell Lea Sugar Free Milk Chocolate can be purchased online at: www.lowcarb outfitters.com.

Remove the pan from the oven and place it on a cooling rack. Cool completely.

To make the Chocolate Coffee Filling, beat the butter in the mixing bowl of an electric mixer on medium speed until light and fluffy. Add ¾ cup Splenda and beat for 3 minutes. Add the chocolate and 1 teaspoon instant coffee and blend well. Add 1 egg and beat for 5 minutes on high speed, scraping down the sides of the bowl with a rubber spatula as necessary. Add the remaining egg and beat for another 5 minutes. Spoon the filling into the cooled crust and smooth the top with a spatula. Refrigerate, covered, for several hours or overnight.

To make the Coffee Topping, combine the whipping cream, ½ tablespoon instant coffee, and ¼ cup Splenda in a chilled bowl. Whip with chilled beaters on medium speed until stiff peaks form. Spread the Coffee Topping over the Chocolate Coffee Filling. Refrigerate until ready to serve.

EACH SERVING PROVIDES:
12g carbohydrates, 307 calories, 4g protein, 28g fat,
1g dietary fiber, 101mg sodium, 84mg cholesterol

Crème Brûlée

This is the perfect dessert to serve after a rich dinner. It is light and flavorful and has the extra distinction of being very low in carbohydrates. To lower the carbohydrates even more in this luscious dessert, simply reduce the brown sugar by half or omit it altogether. If you do not have 4-ounce ramekins, you can use ovenproof coffee cups.

6 SERVINGS

2 cups whipping cream
½ teaspoon vanilla extract
5 large egg yolks

½ cup Splenda
1 tablespoon dark brown sugar
  (optional)

COMBINE the whipping cream and vanilla in a medium saucepan over medium heat. Heat until hot but not boiling. Remove the saucepan from the heat and place it on a cooling rack. Cool slightly. Cover, and refrigerate for 30 minutes.

Preheat oven to 325 degrees F. Place the egg yolks and Splenda in a medium bowl and whisk until well blended. Add the whipping cream mixture and blend well.

Place a small strainer over a 4-ounce ramekin. Pour some whipping cream mixture almost to the top of the dish. Repeat this process with the remaining ramekins. Place the ramekins in a larger pan and put in the oven. Pour enough hot water into the pan to come halfway up the sides of the dishes. Bake for 40 to 50 minutes or until the custards are firm.

Remove the ramekins from the oven and place them on a cooling rack. Cool completely. Cover each Crème Brûlée with a piece of plastic wrap and refrigerate until ready to serve.

(continues)

To serve, uncover the Crème Brûlée and, if desired, sprinkle them with brown sugar, making sure to spread it evenly over the custard.

Preheat the broiler. Place the ramekins on a baking sheet and broil for 1 to 2 minutes or until the sugar begins to caramelize.

EACH SERVING PROVIDES:

5g carbohydrates, 332 calories, 4g protein, 34g fat,
0g dietary fiber, 37mg sodium, 286mg cholesterol

Hazelnut Cake Roll

This ambrosial cake roll can be made with hazelnuts or walnuts, but no matter which ingredient you choose, the light texture, subtly sweet taste, and ease of preparation remain. If you have a craving for chocolate, chocolate shavings made from a ½-ounce bittersweet chocolate square can be sprinkled over the whipped cream filling before rolling it up.

12 SERVINGS

Hazelnut Cake Roll
1⅓ cups toasted hazelnuts
    (filberts), finely chopped*
1 teaspoon baking powder
¼ teaspoon baking soda
¼ teaspoon coarse salt
6 large egg whites, at room
    temperature
6 large egg yolks
¾ cup Splenda

Whipped Cream Filling
1 cup whipping cream
¼ cup Splenda
½ teaspoon vanilla extract
½ ounce semisweet chocolate
    shavings (optional)
½ to 1 teaspoon powdered
    sugar (optional)

PREHEAT oven to 350 degrees F. Lightly coat a 10 × 15-inch jelly-roll pan with a nonstick vegetable spray. Line the pan with a piece of waxed paper and coat again with spray. Set aside.

To make the cake roll, combine the hazelnuts, baking powder, baking soda, and salt in a medium bowl and blend with a wire whisk.

Place the egg whites in the mixing bowl of an electric mixer fitted with the wire whisk attachment and beat on medium-high speed until stiff but not dry. Transfer the whites to a medium bowl.

(continues)

*To toast hazelnuts: Preheat the oven to 350 degrees F, spread the hazelnuts in a single layer in a shallow pan, and bake for 10 minutes or until fragrant.

Place the egg yolks and ¾ cup Splenda in the same mixing bowl. Using the paddle attachment, beat on medium-high speed for 3 minutes. Add the dry ingredients and beat until well blended, scraping down the sides of the bowl with a rubber spatula as necessary. On low speed, add ¼ of the egg whites and beat until just blended. Using a rubber spatula, fold in the remaining egg whites until completely incorporated. Spread the batter in the prepared pan and smooth the top with a spatula. Bake for 15 to 17 minutes or until the top of the cake springs back when lightly touched with a fingertip.

Remove the pan from the oven and place it on a cooling rack. Cover the cake with a piece of waxed paper longer than the cake and then a damp tea towel. Place a cookie sheet over the tea towel and invert the pan and cookie sheet, holding them together as you turn them. Remove the pan and peel off the waxed paper. Quickly roll the cake with the remaining waxed paper and tea towel, starting at the narrow end. Cool completely.

To make the Whipped Cream Filling, place the whipping cream, ¼ cup Splenda, and vanilla in a chilled mixing bowl. Whip with chilled beaters on medium-speed until stiff.

To assemble the cake, place the cake roll on a flat surface and carefully unroll it. Spread the Whipped Cream Filling to the edge on three sides of the cake and almost to the narrow end of the cake. Sprinkle the optional chocolate shavings all over the filling. Reroll the cake, leaving the tea towel and waxed paper behind. Place the cake roll on an oblong cake platter. Cover, and refrigerate for several hours or overnight.

To serve, cut off the ragged edges of the cake on both ends. Place the optional powdered sugar in a fine strainer and dust the top of the cake with it. Using a knife with a serrated edge or a bread knife, cut the Hazelnut Cake Roll into 12 slices.

EACH SERVING PROVIDES:

5g carbohydrates, 209 calories, 5g protein, 19g fat,
1g dietary fiber, 147mg sodium, 133mg cholesterol

Italian Cake Roll

One of my family's favorite recipes is Italian cream cake. Much to our dismay, we found the cake to be a high-carbohydrate disaster. To remedy this, I adapted the original recipe to make it more user friendly.

12 SERVINGS

Italian Cake Roll
1⅓ cups finely chopped pecans
1½ to 2 ounces sweetened coconut
1 teaspoon baking powder
¼ teaspoon baking soda
¼ teaspoon coarse salt
6 large egg whites, at room temperature
6 large egg yolks
¾ cup Splenda

Cream Cheese Filling
1 package (8 ounces) cream cheese, at room temperature
¼ cup (4 tablespoons) butter, at room temperature
½ cup Splenda
¼ cup whipping cream
½ teaspoon vanilla extract
½ to 1 teaspoon powdered sugar (optional)

PREHEAT oven to 350 degrees F. Lightly coat a 10 × 15-inch jelly-roll pan with a nonstick vegetable spray. Line the pan with a piece of waxed paper and coat again with spray. Set aside.

Combine the pecans, coconut, baking powder, baking soda, and salt in a medium bowl and blend with a wire whisk.

To make the cake roll, place the egg whites in the mixing bowl of an electric mixer fitted with the wire whisk attachment and beat on medium-high speed until stiff but not dry. Transfer the whites to a medium bowl.

Place the egg yolks and ¾ cup Splenda in the same mixing bowl. Using the paddle attachment, beat on medium-high speed for 3 minutes.

(continues)

Add the dry ingredients and beat until well blended, scraping down the sides of the bowl with a rubber spatula as necessary. On low speed, add ¼ of the egg whites and beat until just blended. Using a rubber spatula, fold in the remaining egg whites until completely incorporated. Spread the batter in the prepared pan. Smooth the top with a spatula. Bake for 15 to 16 minutes or until the top of the cake springs back when lightly touched with a fingertip.

Remove the pan from the oven and place on a cooling rack. Cover the cake with a piece of waxed paper longer than the cake and then a damp tea towel. Place a cookie sheet over the tea towel and invert the pan and cookie sheet, holding them together as you turn them. Remove the pan and peel off the waxed paper. Quickly roll the cake with the remaining waxed paper and tea towel, starting at the narrow end. Cool completely.

To make the Cream Cheese Filling, place the cream cheese, butter, and ½ cup Splenda in a mixing bowl and beat until light and fluffy. Add the whipping cream and vanilla and beat until well blended.

To assemble the cake, place the cake roll on a flat surface and carefully unroll it. Spread the Cream Cheese Filling to the edge on three sides of the cake and almost to the narrow end of the cake. Reroll the cake, leaving the tea towel and waxed paper behind. Place the cake roll on an oblong cake platter. Cover, and refrigerate for several hours or overnight.

To serve, cut off the ragged edges of the cake on both ends. Place the optional powdered sugar in a fine strainer and dust the top of the cake with it. Using a knife with a serrated edge or a bread knife, cut the Italian Cake Roll into 12 slices.

EACH SERVING PROVIDES:
8g carbohydrates, 270 calories, 6g protein, 25g fat,
1g dietary fiber, 207mg sodium, 144mg cholesterol

Lemon Chiffon Pie

You will adore this light and airy lemon chiffon pie. It has a wonderful subtle, tangy flavor yet is sweet enough to satisfy.

12 SERVINGS

Crust
1 cup high-gluten flour
⅓ cup almond flour
1½ tablespoons Splenda
½ teaspoon coarse salt
2 tablespoons milk
½ cup canola oil

Lemon Chiffon Filling
¼ cup cold water
1 envelope (1 tablespoon)
   unflavored gelatin

4 large egg yolks
1 teaspoon finely grated lemon
   peel
½ cup fresh lemon juice
1 cup Splenda
4 large egg whites, at room
   temperature
⅛ teaspoon coarse salt
1 cup whipping cream

PREHEAT oven to 400 degrees F.
To make the crust, combine the gluten flour, almond flour, 1½ tablespoons Splenda, and salt in a large bowl and blend with a fork. Add the milk and canola oil and mix until well blended. Press the dough into a 9-inch pie pan. Bake for 10 minutes.

Remove the pan from the oven and place on a cooling rack.

To make the Lemon Chiffon Filling, pour the cold water in a small dish. Sprinkle the gelatin over the water. Set aside.

Place the egg yolks in the top of a double boiler and blend. Add the lemon peel. Gradually add the lemon juice and ½ cup Splenda, stirring constantly. Place over hot water and cook until mixture thickens slightly or registers 175 to 180 degrees F on a candy thermometer. Remove

(continues)

Dazzling Desserts
••••

the top from the heat and add the gelatin. Stir until the gelatin has dissolved. Cool completely, stirring occasionally.

Place the egg whites and salt in the mixing bowl of an electric mixer fitted with the wire whisk attachment (or use a hand-held beater) and beat until soft peaks form. Gradually add the remaining ½ cup Splenda and beat until stiff. Transfer the egg whites to a clean bowl.

Place the whipping cream in a chilled mixing bowl. Beat with chilled beaters until soft peaks form.

Using a rubber spatula, gradually fold the lemon mixture into the egg whites. Fold in the whipped cream until fully incorporated. Spoon the Lemon Chiffon Filling into the prepared crust. Refrigerate for several hours or overnight.

EACH SERVING PROVIDES:
12g carbohydrates, 243 calories, 5g protein, 20g fat,
1g dietary fiber, 131mg sodium, 98mg cholesterol

Panna Cotta

A panna cotta is the ultimate low-carbohydrate dessert. Translated from Italian, it literally means "cooked cream." Actually, it is barely cooked—just enough to dissolve the gelatin. The final result tastes like vanilla pudding and has the texture of an "upscale" Jell-O mold. You can serve this scrumptious dessert alone, or it can be garnished with fresh raspberries or sliced strawberries.

8 SERVINGS

½ cup milk
2 teaspoons unflavored gelatin
1½ cups whipping cream
1 vanilla bean, 2 inches long and slit lengthwise (or 1 tablespoon vanilla extract)

¼ cup Splenda
Scant ⅛ teaspoon coarse salt
1 cup raspberries or sliced strawberries, for garnish
8 sprigs fresh mint, for garnish

LIGHTLY coat eight 4-ounce ramekins (or small coffee cups) with a nonstick vegetable spray.

Pour the milk in a small saucepan and sprinkle the gelatin over the top. Allow it to stand for 5 to 10 minutes or until the gelatin softens.

In the meantime, prepare an ice bath by filling a large bowl with ice cubes and cold water. Set aside.

Place the whipping cream in a medium bowl. Lay the vanilla bean flat and use a paring knife to split the bean lengthwise. Using the dull side of the knife, scrape the seeds from the vanilla bean into the whipping cream and lightly blend. Set aside.

Heat the milk and gelatin mixture over high heat and cook for 1 to 2 minutes or until a candy thermometer registers 135 degrees F, stirring constantly. Remove the saucepan from the heat and add the Splenda and salt; blend well. Gradually add the whipping cream

(continues)

mixture, stirring constantly. Set the saucepan in the ice water for 5 to 10 minutes or until it is the consistency of lightly beaten whipped cream, stirring occasionally.

Pour the whipping cream mixture into the prepared ramekins, dividing evenly. Refrigerate for several hours or overnight.

To serve, fill a small bowl with boiling water. Dip each ramekin in the water for 2 to 4 seconds to loosen the mold. Remove the ramekin from the water and use your fingertips to press lightly around the edges of the Panna Cotta. Dip the ramekin in the water for another 2 to 4 seconds. Quickly wipe the bottom of the ramekin with a towel and place a dessert plate over the top and invert. Remove the ramekin and garnish each serving with fruit and a sprig of mint, if desired.

EACH SERVING PROVIDES:
3g carbohydrates, 168 calories, 2g protein, 17g fat,
0g dietary fiber, 55mg sodium, 63mg cholesterol

ABOUT VANILLA BEANS

A vanilla bean imparts an intensely rich and pure vanilla flavor. Much of the intense flavor is derived from the seeds or the dark, sticky pulp found within the vanilla bean. When choosing a vanilla bean, look for a long, plump one that is pliable and, at the same time, feels dense and squishy. If you can smell the vanilla bean, it should have a characteristic vanilla fragrance.

Pecan Torte

This torte is a perfect dessert or a deliciously sweet indulgence to serve after the movies. It is composed of a pecan cake covered with a delectable whipped cream topping and can be crowned with a layer of semisweet chocolate shavings.

12 SERVINGS

Pecan Cake
7 large egg whites, at room temperature
¼ cup Splenda
7 large egg yolks
1 cup finely chopped pecans
¼ cup chopped peeled apple
2 tablespoons almond flour
1 teaspoon finely grated lemon peel

1 teaspoon vanilla extract
½ teaspoon powdered white stevia

Whipped Cream Topping
¾ cup whipping cream
1½ tablespoons Splenda
½ teaspoon vanilla extract
Semisweet chocolate shavings (optional)

PREHEAT oven to 350 degrees F. Lightly coat an 8-inch springform pan with a nonstick vegetable spray. Cut an 8-inch round of waxed paper and line the bottom of the pan with it. Spray again.

To make the pecan cake, place the egg whites in the mixing bowl of an electric mixer fitted with the wire whisk attachment and beat on medium-high speed until soft peaks form. Gradually add ¼ cup Splenda and beat until firm but not dry. Transfer the whites to a medium bowl.

Place the egg yolks, pecans, apple, almond flour, lemon peel, 1 teaspoon vanilla, and stevia in the mixing bowl. Using the paddle attachment, beat until well blended. Using a rubber spatula, fold ¼ of the egg whites into the egg yolk mixture to lighten it. Add the remaining egg whites and gently fold until completely incorporated. Spoon the

(continues)

batter into the prepared pan and smooth the top with a rubber spatula. Bake for 30 to 35 minutes or until a cake tester inserted into the center of the cake comes out clean.

Remove the pan from the oven and place on a cooling rack. Cover with waxed paper and cool completely. When cool, remove the waxed paper and the sides of the springform pan. Invert the cake onto a cake plate and remove the waxed paper round.

To make the Whipped Cream Topping, place the whipping cream, 1½ tablespoons Splenda, and ½ teaspoon vanilla in a chilled mixing bowl. Whip with chilled beaters on medium speed until stiff.

To assemble the torte, place strips of waxed paper under the edges of the cake to keep the Whipped Cream Topping off the plate. Using a metal spatula, spread the Whipped Cream Topping over the top and sides of the cake. Sprinkle the top of the torte with the chocolate shavings, if desired. Remove the strips of wax paper. The torte can be served immediately or refrigerated for several hours or overnight.

EACH SERVING PROVIDES:
5g carbohydrates, 178 calories, 5g protein, 16g fat,
1g dietary fiber, 43mg sodium, 144mg cholesterol

Pumpkin Cake Roll

This light and airy dessert is a sensational combination of spice-laced pumpkin cake filled with a rich cream cheese frosting. If your taste runs toward whipped cream fillings (in Hazelnut Cake Roll on page 365), then simply substitute it for the cream cheese recipe.

12 SERVINGS

Pumpkin Cake Roll
½ cup vanilla whey protein powder
¼ cup almond flour
2 teaspoons ground cinnamon
1 teaspoon ground ginger
1 teaspoon ground nutmeg
1 teaspoon baking powder
1 teaspoon baking soda
¼ teaspoon coarse salt
3 large eggs
¾ cup Splenda
1 teaspoon powdered white stevia

⅔ cup solid-packed pumpkin
1 teaspoon fresh lemon juice

Cream Cheese Filling*
1 package (8 ounces) cream cheese, at room temperature
¼ cup (4 tablespoons) butter, at room temperature
½ cup Splenda
¼ cup whipping cream
½ teaspoon vanilla extract (optional)
½ to 1 teaspoon powdered sugar (optional)

PREHEAT oven to 350 degrees F. Lightly coat a 10 × 15-inch jelly-roll pan with a nonstick vegetable spray. Line the pan with a piece of waxed paper and coat again with spray. Set aside.

To make the Pumpkin Cake Roll, combine the protein powder, almond flour, cinnamon, ginger, nutmeg, baking powder, baking soda, and salt in a medium bowl and blend with a wire whisk.

(continues)

*To reduce the fat and calorie content in the Cream Cheese Filling, use 6 tablespoons cream cheese, 3 tablespoons butter, 6 tablespoons Splenda, 3 tablespoons whipping cream, and ½ teaspoon vanilla extract.

Place the eggs, ¾ cup Splenda, and stevia in the mixing bowl of an electric mixer and beat on medium-high speed for 5 minutes. Add the pumpkin and lemon juice and blend well. On medium-low speed, slowly add the dry ingredients and beat until just blended. Spread the batter in the prepared pan and smooth the top with a spatula. Bake for 8 to 10 minutes or until the top of the cake springs back when lightly touched with a fingertip.

Remove the pan from the oven and place on a cooling rack. Cover the cake with a piece of waxed paper longer than the cake and then a damp tea towel. Place a cookie sheet over the tea towel and invert the pan and cookie sheet, holding them together as you turn them. Remove the pan and peel off the waxed paper. Quickly roll the cake with the remaining waxed paper and tea towel, starting at the narrow end. Cool completely.

To make the Cream Cheese Filling, place the cream cheese, butter, and ½ cup Splenda in a mixing bowl and beat until light and fluffy. Add the whipping cream and optional vanilla and beat until well blended.

To assemble the cake, place the cake roll on a flat surface and carefully unroll it. Spread the Cream Cheese Filling to the edge on three sides of the cake and almost to the narrow end of the cake. Reroll the cake, leaving the tea towel and waxed paper behind. Place the cake roll on an oblong cake platter. Cover, and refrigerate for several hours or overnight.

To serve, cut off the ragged edges of the cake on both ends. Place the powdered sugar in a fine strainer and dust the top of the cake with it, if desired. Using a knife with a serrated edge or a bread knife, cut the Pumpkin Cake Roll into 12 slices.

EACH SERVING PROVIDES:
6g carbohydrates, 185 calories, 7g protein, 15g fat,
1g dietary fiber, 270mg sodium, 97mg cholesterol

Pumpkin Cheesecake

A delicately spiced pumpkin cheesecake is a lovely finale to a holiday dinner. It is delicious when topped with a dollop of ginger-flavored whipped cream.

12 TO 16 SERVINGS

Walnut Crust
½ cup walnuts

Cheesecake Filling
3 packages (8 ounces each)
    cream cheese, at room
    temperature
1 cup Splenda
1 teaspoon powdered white
    stevia

1 teaspoon ground cinnamon
⅛ teaspoon ground ginger
⅛ teaspoon ground cardamom
⅛ teaspoon ground nutmeg
⅛ teaspoon ground cloves
¼ cup whipping cream
2 teaspoons vanilla extract
3 large eggs
¾ cup solid-packed pumpkin

PREHEAT oven to 350 degrees F. Lightly coat a 9-inch springform pan with a nonstick vegetable spray.

To make the Walnut Crust, place the walnuts in the work bowl of a food processor fitted with a metal blade (or in a blender) and pulse until finely chopped. Press the walnuts on the bottom of the prepared pan. Bake for 5 minutes.

Remove the pan from the oven and place on a cooling rack. Cool completely.

To make the filling, place the cream cheese, Splenda, and stevia in the mixing bowl of an electric mixer and beat on medium-high speed for 3 minutes, scraping down the sides of the bowl with a rubber spatula as necessary. Add the cinnamon, ginger, cardamom, nutmeg, and cloves and blend well. On medium speed, add the whipping cream

(continues)

and vanilla and beat for 2 minutes. Add the eggs, one at a time, beating well after each addition and scraping down the sides of the bowl. Add the pumpkin and beat until thoroughly combined. Pour the batter into the prepared pan. Place the pan in a larger pan and put in the oven. Pour enough hot water into the pan to come halfway up the sides of the pan. Bake for 60 minutes.

Turn off the oven heat and open the door slightly. Leave the cheesecake in the oven for 1 hour. Remove the cheesecake from the oven, cover, and refrigerate for several hours or overnight.

VARIATION: To make Ginger-Flavored Whipped Cream, place 1 cup whipping cream, 2 tablespoons Splenda, and ½ teaspoon ground ginger in a chilled mixing bowl. Whip with chilled beaters on medium speed until stiff.

EACH SERVING PROVIDES:
6g carbohydrates, 281 calories, 7g protein, 26g fat,
1g dietary fiber, 188mg sodium, 122mg cholesterol

Pumpkin Custard

After enjoying a festive dinner, you will delight in the richly sweet and flavorful satisfaction of this upscale dessert. The custard is also delicious without the addition of the brown sugar topping, so to shave some calories, feel free to omit it or reduce the amount by half.

6 SERVINGS

1 cup whipping cream
1 cup milk
5 tablespoons Splenda
1 2-inch cinnamon stick
¼ teaspoon ground allspice
⅛ teaspoon ground ginger
⅛ teaspoon ground cloves

⅛ teaspoon ground nutmeg
4 large egg yolks
6 tablespoons solid-packed pumpkin
1 tablespoon dark brown sugar (optional)

COMBINE the whipping cream, milk, Splenda, cinnamon stick, allspice, ginger, cloves, and nutmeg in a medium saucepan over medium heat. Heat until hot but not boiling.

Remove the saucepan from the heat and place it on a cooling rack. Cool slightly. Cover, and refrigerate for 30 minutes.

Preheat oven to 350 degrees F. Remove the cinnamon stick from the whipping cream mixture. Add the egg yolks and beat with a wire whisk until smooth. Add the pumpkin and whisk until well blended and smooth.

Place a small strainer over a 4-ounce ramekin. Pour the pumpkin mixture almost to the top of the dish. Repeat this process with the remaining ramekins. Place the ramekins in a larger pan and put in the oven. Pour enough hot water into the pan to come halfway up the sides of the dishes. Bake for 35 to 40 minutes or until the custards are firm and a knife inserted into the center comes out clean.

(continues)

Remove the ramekins from the oven and place them on a cooling rack. When cool, cover each with a piece of plastic wrap and refrigerate for several hours or overnight.

To serve, uncover the pumpkin custard and sprinkle them with dark brown sugar, if desired, making sure it is spread evenly over the custard. Preheat the broiler, place the ramekins on a baking sheet, and broil for 30 to 60 seconds or until the sugar begins to caramelize.

EACH SERVING PROVIDES:

6g carbohydrates, 212 calories, 4g protein, 20g fat,
0g dietary fiber, 42mg sodium, 202mg cholesterol

The Ultimate Cheesecake

If you love the rich flavor and creamy texture of a traditional cheesecake, you'll be amazed to find out that this low-carb version is as satisfying as the sinfully high-carb original. I often add a sour cream layer after the cheesecake is almost done baking, but it is not necessary. If your low-carb diet allows fruit, then a topping of fresh strawberries or blueberries would be a nice way to crown the dessert.

12 TO 16 SERVINGS

Walnut Crust
½ cup walnuts

Cheesecake Filling
3 packages (8 ounces each)
   cream cheese, at room
   temperature
¾ cup Splenda
1 teaspoon powdered white
   stevia

4 large eggs
1½ teaspoons vanilla extract
¼ cup whipping cream

Sour Cream Topping (optional)
1 cup sour cream
1 tablespoon Splenda
½ teaspoon vanilla extract

PREHEAT oven to 350 degrees F. Lightly coat a 9-inch springform pan with a nonstick vegetable spray.

To make the Walnut Crust, place the walnuts in the work bowl of a food processor fitted with a metal blade (or in a blender) and pulse until finely chopped. Press the walnuts on the bottom of the prepared pan. Bake for 5 minutes.

Remove the pan from the oven and place on a cooling rack. Cool completely.

(continues)

To make the filling, place the cream cheese, ¾ cup Splenda, and stevia in the mixing bowl of an electric mixer and beat on medium-high speed for 3 minutes, scraping down the sides of the bowl with a rubber spatula as necessary. Add the eggs and 1½ teaspoons vanilla and beat well. On medium speed, add the whipping cream and beat for 2 minutes. Pour the batter into the pan. Place the pan in a larger pan and put in the oven. Pour enough hot water into the pan to come halfway up the sides of the pan. Bake for 45 minutes.

To make the Sour Cream Topping, combine the sour cream, 1 tablespoon Splenda, and ½ teaspoon vanilla in a small bowl and blend well. Remove the cheesecake from the oven and cool for at least 5 minutes. Spread the Sour Cream Topping over the top of the cheesecake. Bake for 5 minutes.

With or without the topping, turn off the oven at the allotted time and open the oven door slightly. Leave the cheesecake in the oven for 1 hour. Remove the cheesecake from the oven, cover, and refrigerate for several hours or overnight.

EACH SERVING PROVIDES:
5g carbohydrates, 320 calories, 8g protein, 30g fat,
0g dietary fiber, 202mg sodium, 157mg cholesterol

READING RESOURCES

The Carbohydrate Addict's LifeSpan Program, Richard F. Heller, M.S., Ph.D., and Rachael F. Heller, M.A., Ph.D., (New York: Dutton, 1995).

Dr. Atkins' New Diet Revolution, Robert C. Atkins, M.D., (New York: Avon, 1992).

Protein Power, Michael R.Eades, M.D., and Mary Dan Eades, M.D., (New York: Bantam, 1996).

Sugar Busters!, H. Leighton Steward et al., (New York: Ballantine, 1998).

The Zone, Barry Sears, Ph.D., (New York: Harper Collins, 1995).

INDEX

Index
••••

International Conversion Chart

These are not exact equivalents: they have been slightly rounded to make measuring easier.

LIQUID MEASUREMENTS

American	Imperial	Metric	Australian
2 tablespoons (1 oz.)	1 fl. oz.	30 ml	1 tablespoon
¼ cup (2 oz.)	2 fl. oz.	60 ml	2 tablespoons
⅓ cup (3 oz.)	3 fl. oz.	80 ml	¼ cup
½ cup (4 oz.)	4 fl. oz.	125 ml	⅓ cup
⅔ cup (5 oz.)	5 fl. oz.	165 ml	½ cup
¾ cup (6 oz.)	6 fl. oz.	185 ml	⅔ cup
1 cup (8 oz.)	8 fl. oz.	250 ml	¾ cup

SPOON MEASUREMENTS

American	Metric
¼ teaspoon	1 ml
½ teaspoon	2 ml
1 teaspoon	5 ml
1 tablespoon	15 ml

WEIGHTS

US/UK	Metric
1 oz.	30 grams (g)
2 oz.	60 g
4 oz. (¼ lb)	125 g
5 oz. (⅓ lb)	155 g
6 oz.	185 g
7 oz.	220 g
8 oz. (½ lb)	250 g
10 oz.	315 g
12 oz. (¾ lb)	375 g
14 oz.	440 g
16 oz. (1 lb)	500 g
2 lbs	1 kg

OVEN TEMPERATURES

Farenheit	Centigrade	Gas
250	120	½
300	150	2
325	160	3
350	180	4
375	190	5
400	200	6
450	230	8